C000318446

LITTLE BOOK OF

YOGA

LITTLE BOOK OF

YOGA

First published in the UK in 2013

© Demand Media Limited 2014

www.demand-media.co.uk

All rights reserved. No part of this work may be reproduced or utilised in any form or by any means, electronic or mechanical, including photocopying, recording or by any information storage and retrieval system, without prior written permission of the publisher.

Printed and bound in Europe.

ISBN 978-1-782811-80-0

The views in this book are those of the author but they are general views only and readers are urged to consult the relevant and qualified specialist for individual advice in particular situations.

Demand Media Limited hereby exclude all liability to the extent permitted by law of any errors or omissions in this book and for any loss, damage or expense (whether direct or indirect) suffered by a third party relying on any information contained in this book.

All our best endeavours have been made to secure copyright clearance for every photograph used but in the event of any copyright owner being overlooked please address correspondence to Demand Media Limited, Waterside Chambers, Bridge Barn Lane, Woking, Surrey, GU21 6NL

In no way will Demand Media Limited or any persons associated with Demand Media be held responsible for any injuries or problems that may occur during the use of this book or the advise contained within. We recommend that you consult a doctor before embarking any exercise programme. This product is for informational purposes only and is not meant as medical advice. Performing exercise of all types can pose a risk, know your physical limits, we suggest you perform adequate warm up and cool downs before and after any exercise. If you experience any pain, discomfort, dizziness or become short of breath stop exercising immediately and consult your doctor.

Contents

Introduction

Originating in ancient India, yoga is a commonly known generic term for the physical, mental and spiritual practices or disciplines that have the sole aim of creating a state of permanent peace. Yoga, specifically, is one of the six orthodox schools of Hindu philosophy. Different traditions of yoga can be found also in Buddhism, Jainism and Sikhism.

Hindu monks brought yoga, particularly what is known as Hatha yoga, to the western world in the late 19th century and it became a popular method of physical exercise during the 1980s.

Apart from the spiritual goals, the physical postures of yoga are used to alleviate health problems, reduce stress and make the spine supple in contemporary times. Yoga is also used as a complete exercise programme and physical therapy routine.

Pilates is a physical fitness system developed in the early 20th century by Joseph Pilates whose concept was intended to strengthen the human mind and body. Pilates believed that mental and physical health is interrelated. It is an extremely popular method of exercise all over the world. Pilates called his method 'Contrology' from the word 'control'.

The techniques employed for pilates builds up flexibility, muscle strength, and endurance in the legs, abdominals, arms, hips and back. It puts emphasis on spinal and pelvic alignment, breathing and developing a strong core, as well as improving coordination and balance. The pilates' method allows for different exercises to be modified in range of difficulty from beginner to advanced. Intensity of exercises can therefore be increased over time as the body conditions and adapts to the exercises.

Yoga and pilates is for inner strength and outer radiance.

The exercises here have been carefully selected by Maddy Barrington-Groves (pictured throughout) and are a fusion of the best aspects of yoga and pilates. They will build up core strength, improve posture, improve flexibility and range of movement, and stretches will tease out tension from the body and ease away aches and pains.

Exercises should be performed slowly and mindfully to rebalance the nervous system, to centre the mind and to increase body awareness. From regular practice, you will look and feel taller, slimmer and more confident, not to mention becoming more at ease in body and mind. You will feel more energy, vitality, and will experience more clarity of thought.

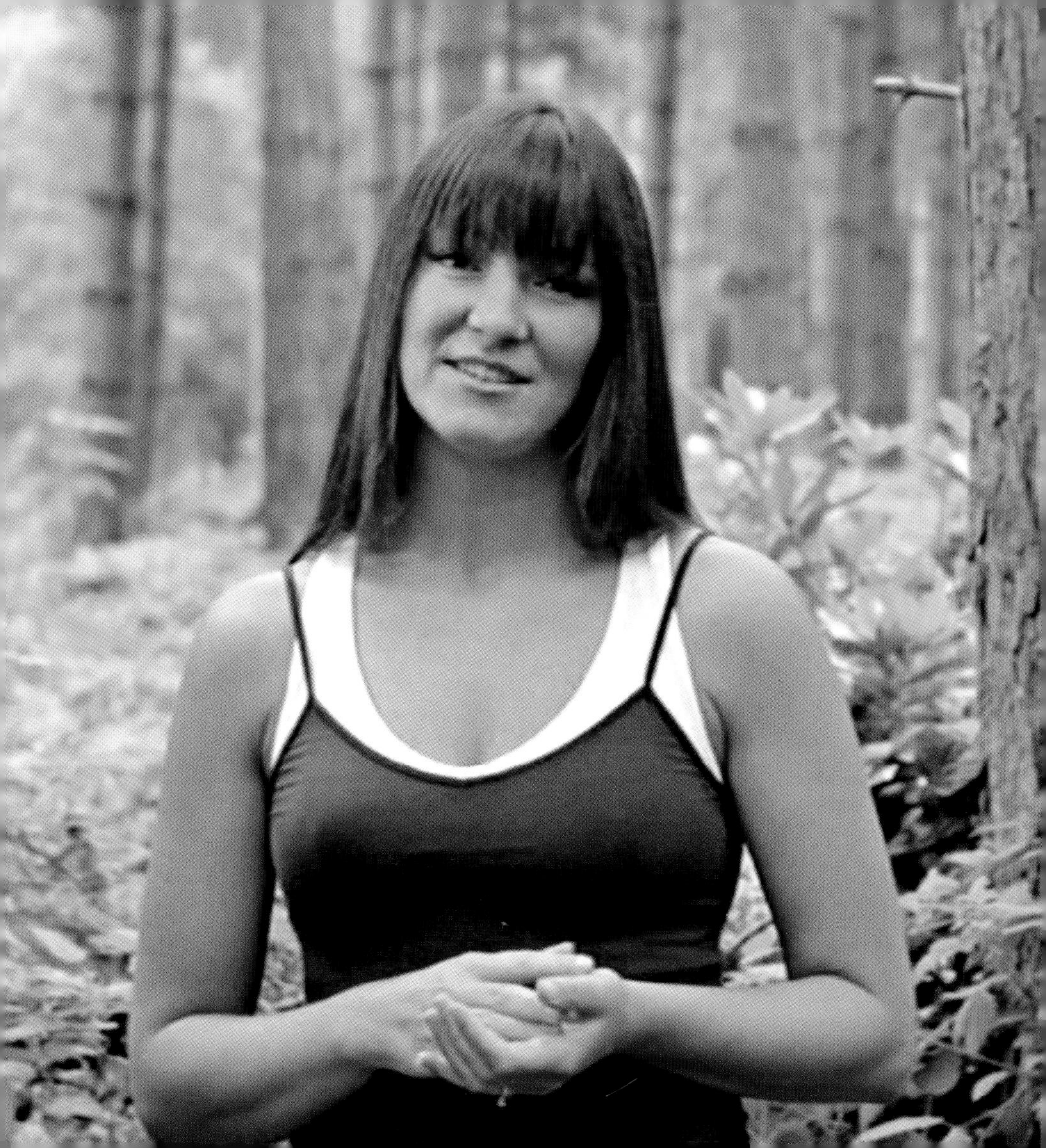

Chapter 1

Engaging the Core and Limbering Up

Stand on the mat with your feet hip width apart with feet parallel.

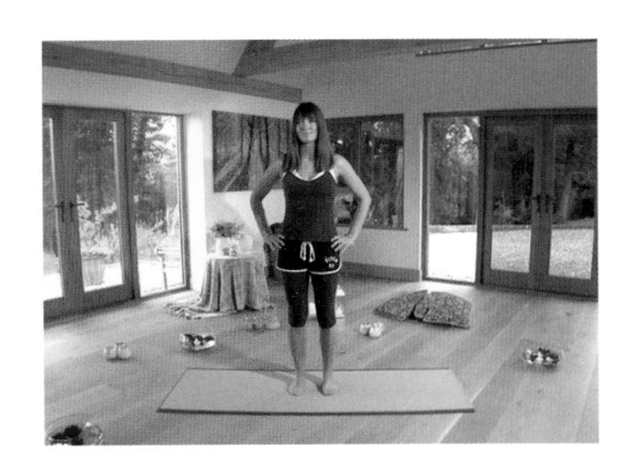

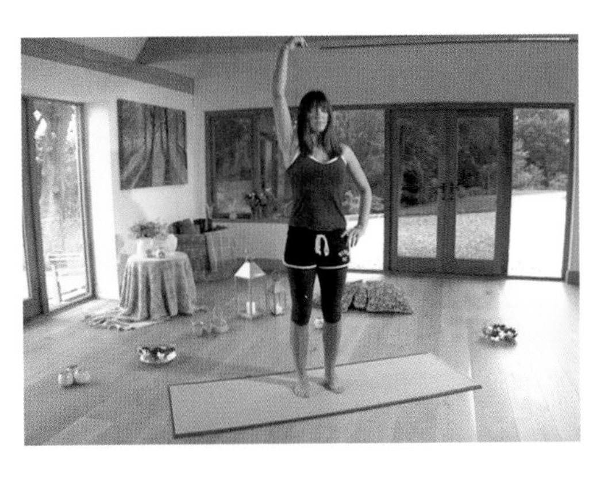

Engage the front of the thighs by lifting up on the kneecaps, lengthening through the spine standing tall, reaching up through the crown of your head.

Bring the hands onto the hips and tilt the pelvis backwards and forwards until a neutral spine position is found. Make sure the pelvis isn't tilted too far either way – it has to be nice and even.

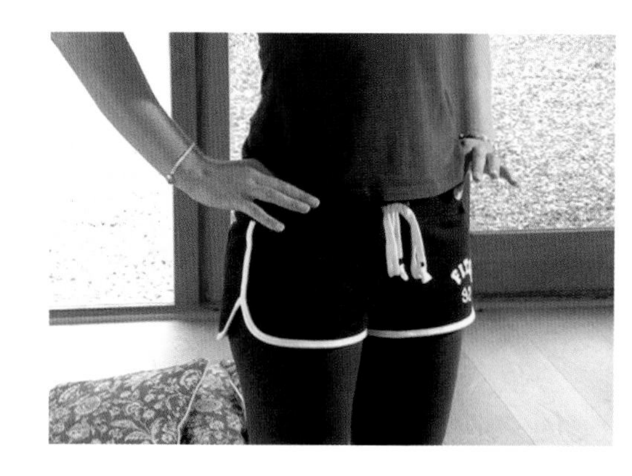

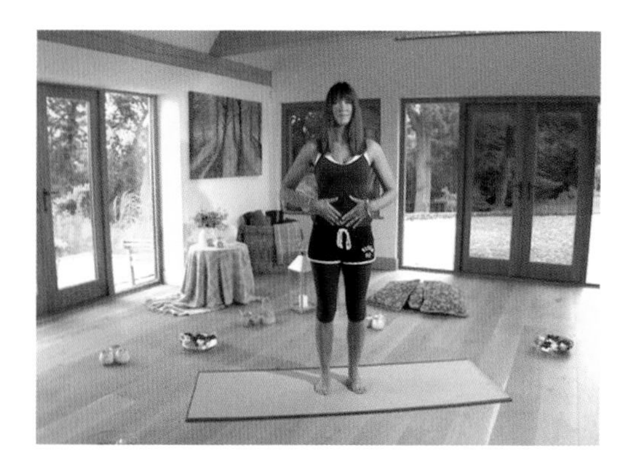

To engage the core as you breath: balloon out your belly as you inhale drawing the navel and stomach muscles back towards the spine as you exhale. Repeat this, but each time reduce the amount of contraction of stomach muscles from 100% to 50% then to 30%.

Hold them at 30% and take several long deep breaths in and out breathing each time right up into the chest. Engage the stomach muscles and pelvic floor every time you breathe up into the chest. The deep core muscles around the pelvis are engaged and the core muscles around the stomach and lower back are engaged as well. It should be a light engaging of the muscles, not a really strong contraction.

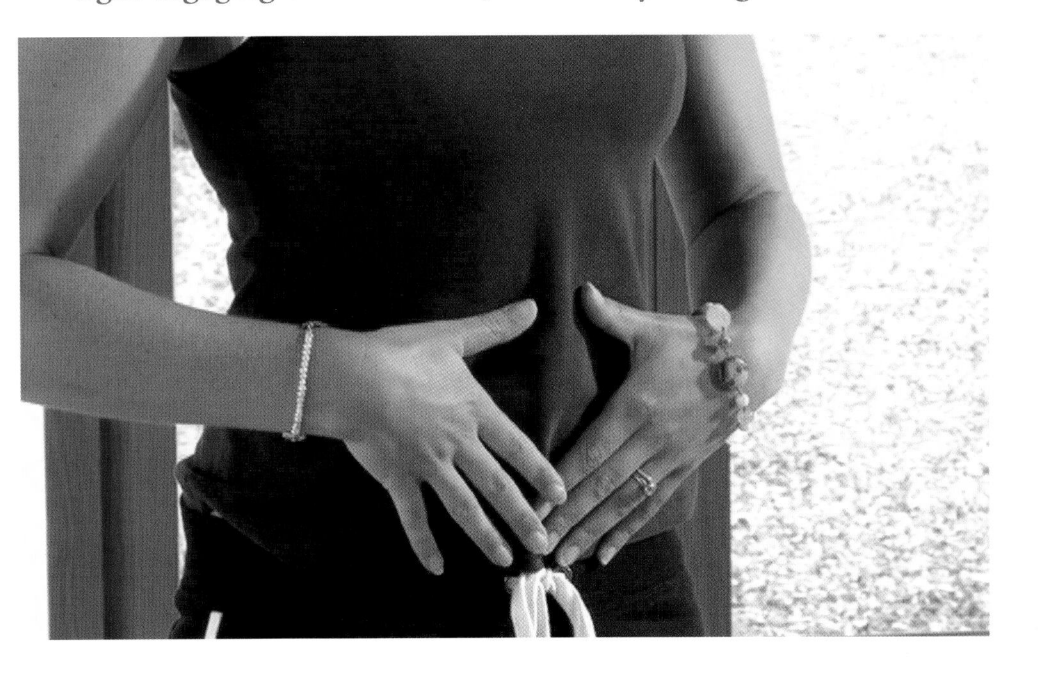

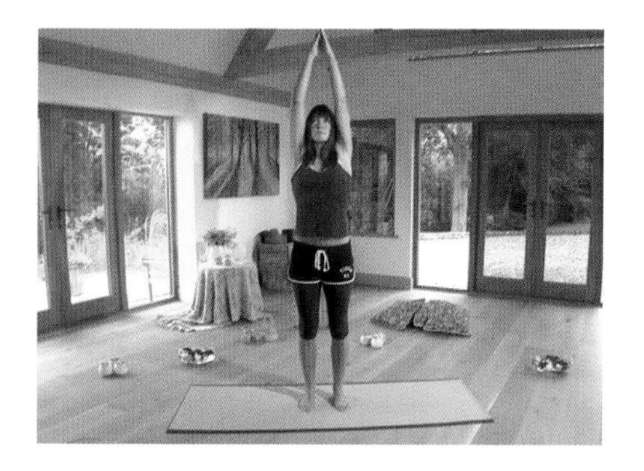

Inhale raising your arms up bringing the palms of your hands together and stretching high.

Then release the arms down. Repeat this twice more.

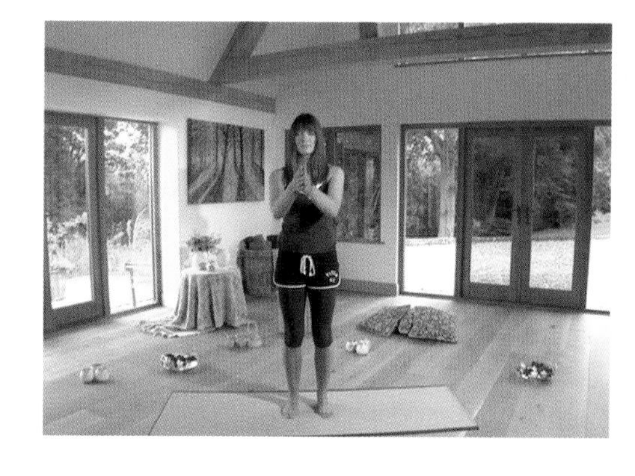

Step 1

Raise the arms up, and holding onto one wrist, stretch over to one side.

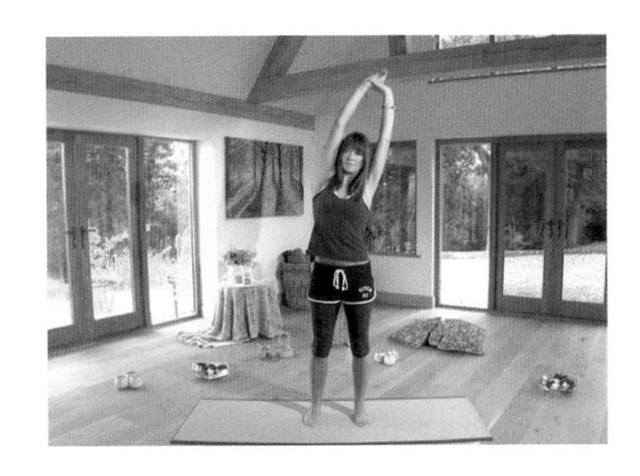

Step 2

Then holding onto the other wrist, stretch over to the other side.

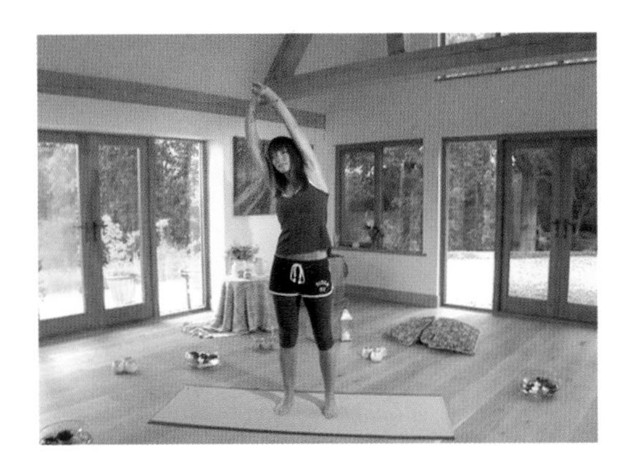

Release the arms back to centre and then bring the arms back down.

Inhale raising the arms up and moving into a full body circle, circling the body all the way round, reaching up through the fingers and circling round folding forward letting the head relax at the bottom. Repeat four times.

Step 1

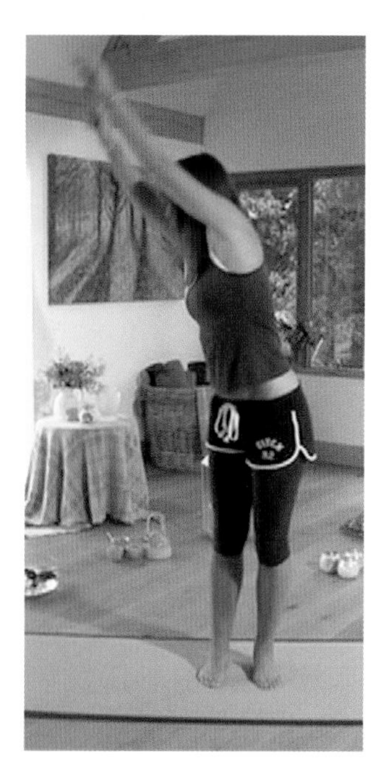

Step 2

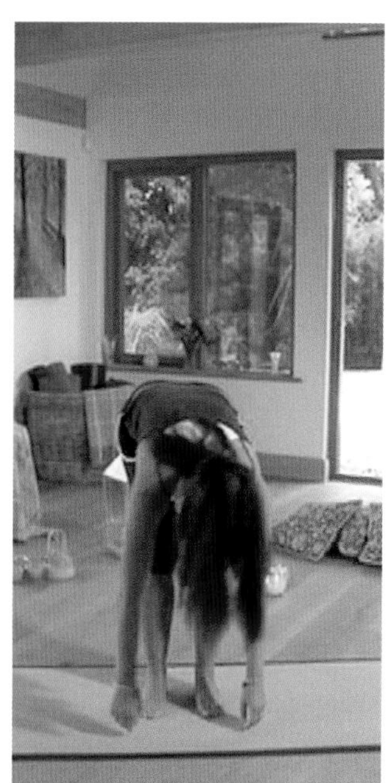

Step 3

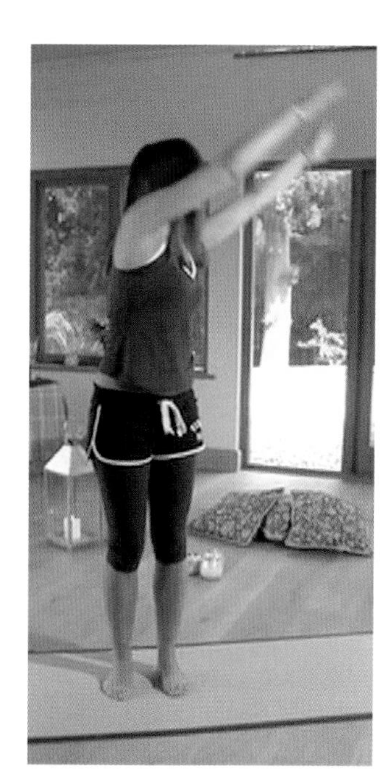

Repeat the exercise circling the other way. Release back to centre, stretching high and then releasing the arms down.

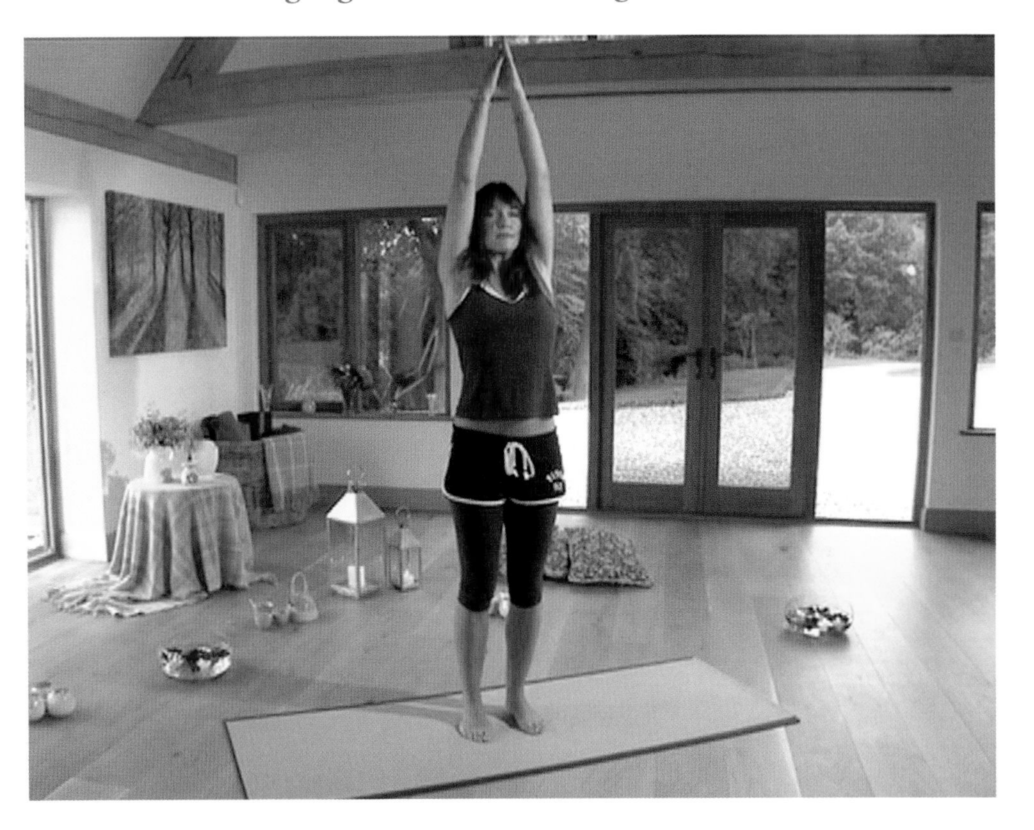

Step 1

Move into roll downs – tuck the chin under.

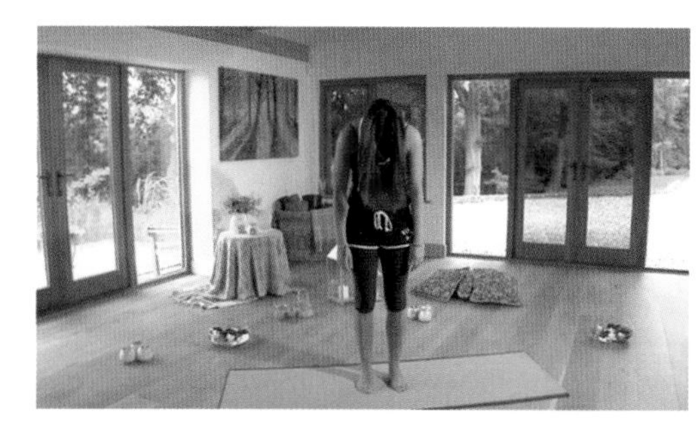

Step 2

Let the sternum and chest soften, let the head and shoulders relax.

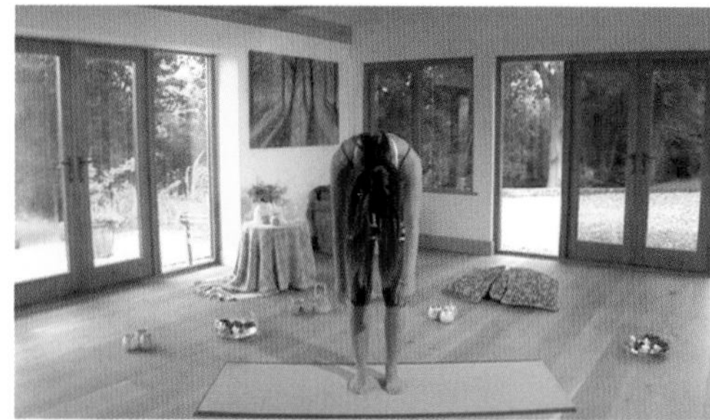

Step 3

Gently roll down, vertebra by vertebra.

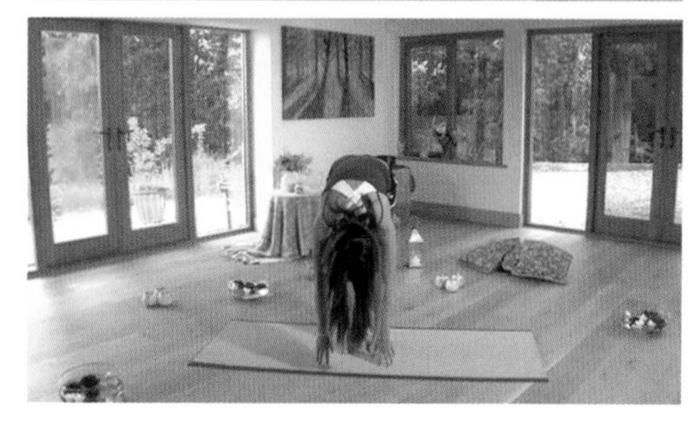

Bending the knees slightly, stretch out one leg at a time by bending one knee and then the other, letting the head and arms relax.

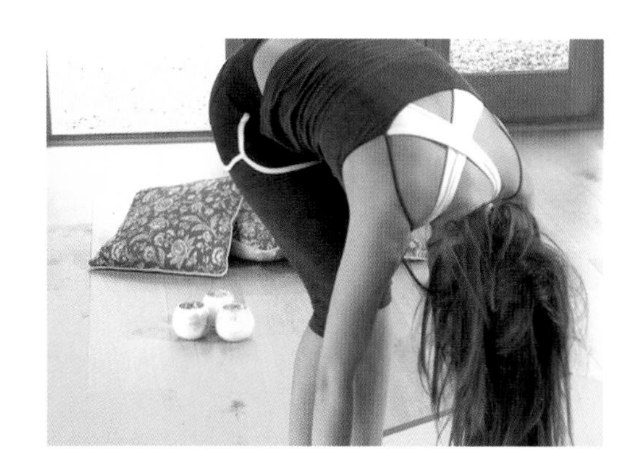

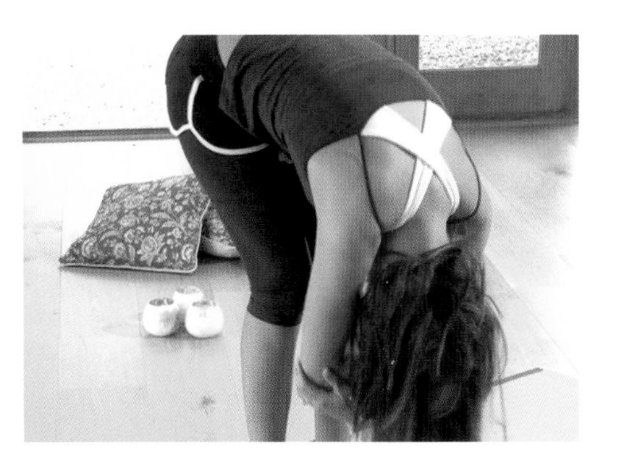

Holding onto the elbows, let the upper body hang heavy; soften the knees.

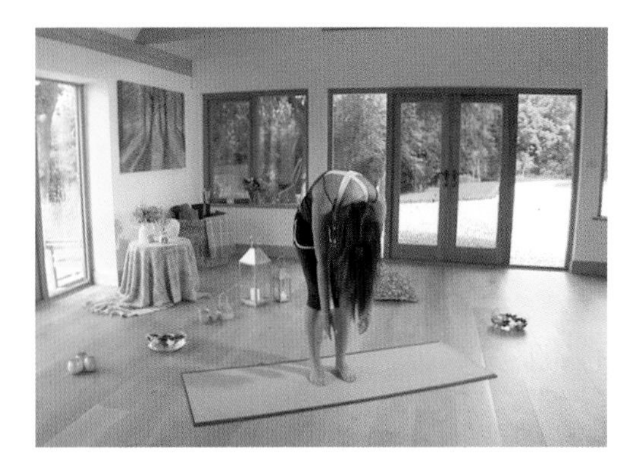

Inhale, and as you exhale begin to unravel, uncurling the spine.

Bring the palms together stretching high, then release your arms down beside you and shake out your shoulders.

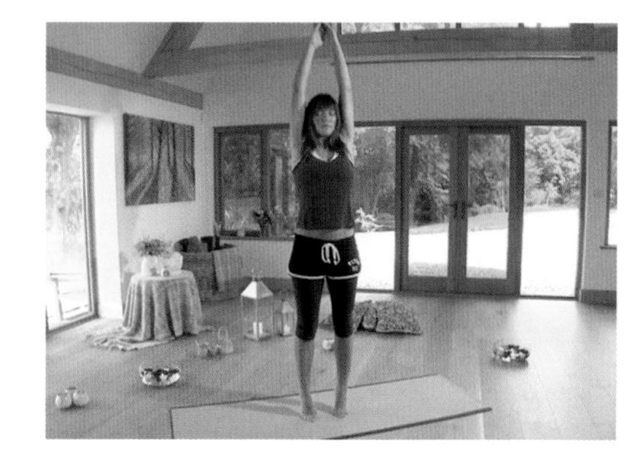

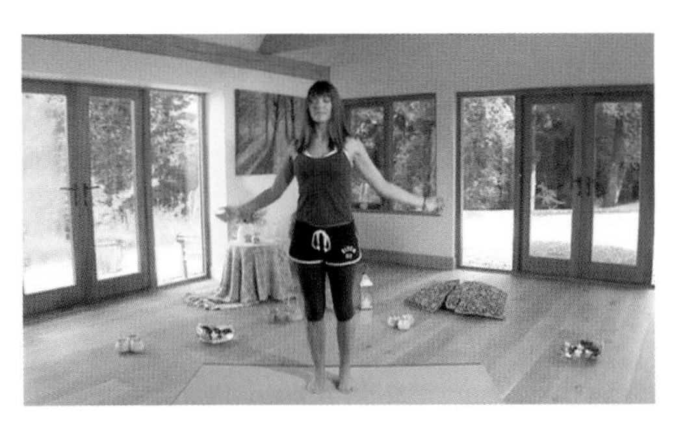

Roll the shoulders back a few times doing nice loose relaxed shoulder rolls.

Hunch the shoulders up around the ears, then draw the shoulders back around the back and relax.

Step 1

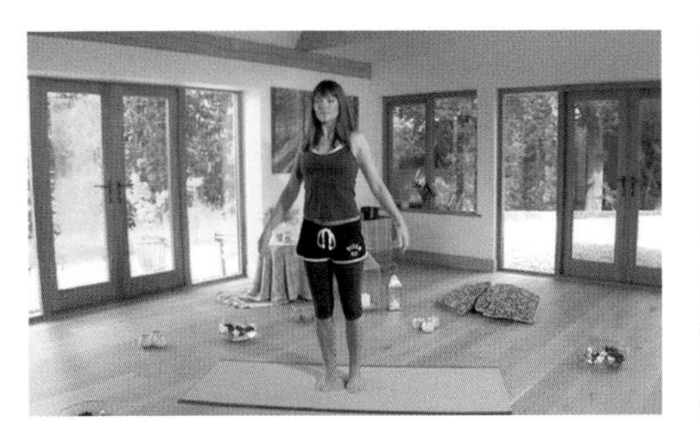

Step 2

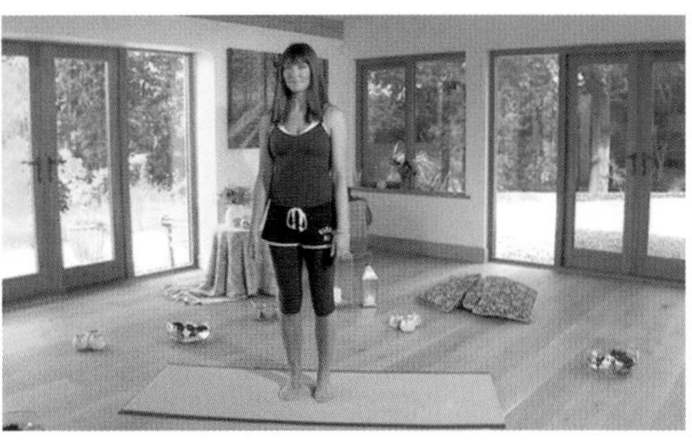

Chapter 2

Toning the Abdominals and Shaping the Waist

Lie down on the floor in a comfortable position, making yourself as long as possible. Bring your arms back behind moving into a full body stretch, reaching through the fingers and toes.

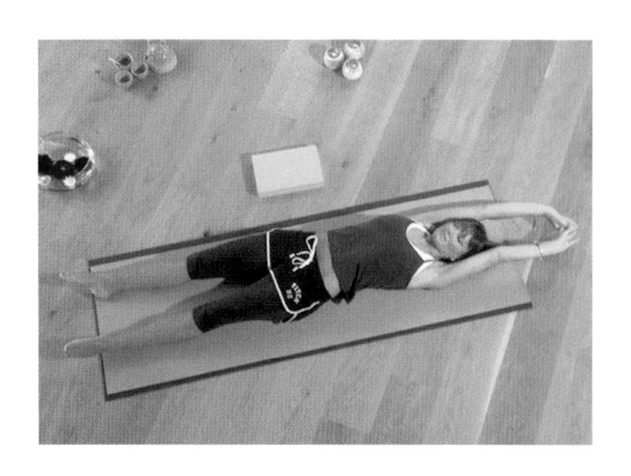

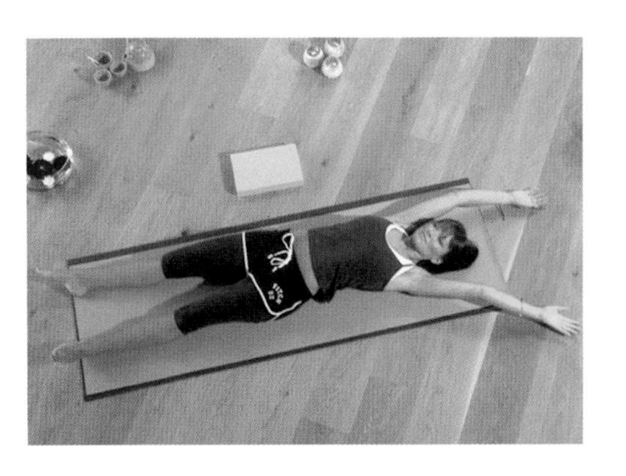

Reach with the right arm and the left leg and then the left arm and the right leg for a diagonal stretch across.

Hold onto the right wrist stretching out the right side then holding onto the left wrist to do the same on the other side.

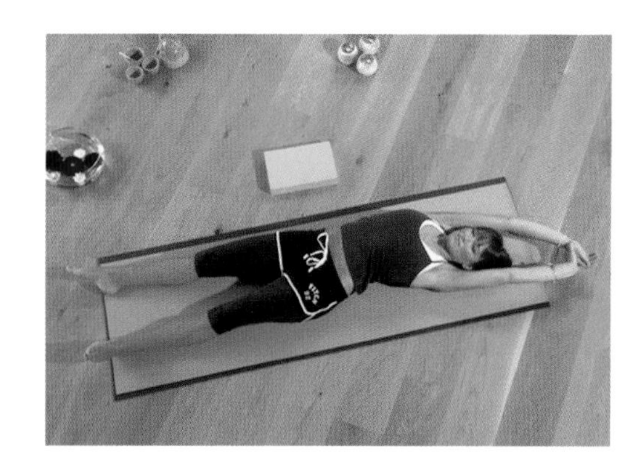

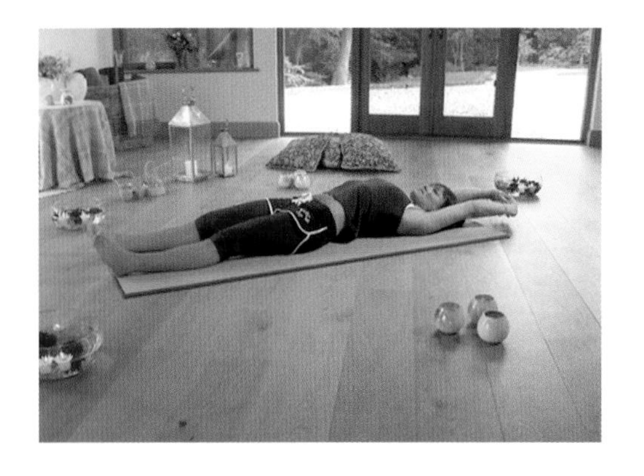

Interlace the hands and stretch out with them above your head.

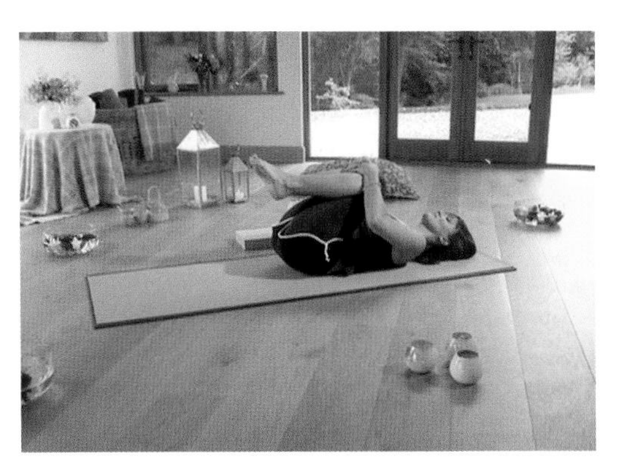

Release the arms and bring your knees up to your chest, hugging them in, then rock gently side to side.

Begin to circle the knees around in small circles, loosening up the lower back. Then circle the other way, stretching out the back.

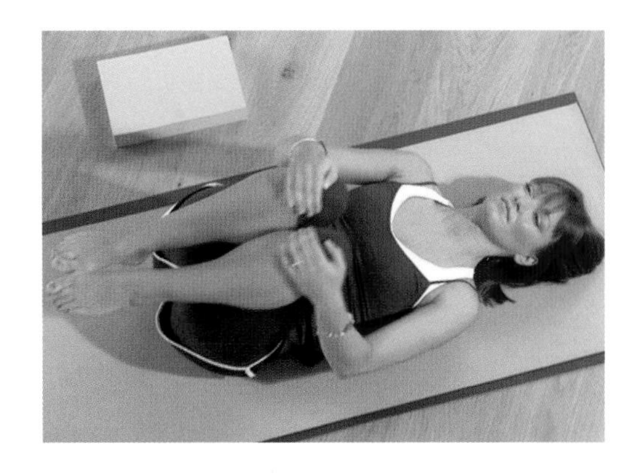

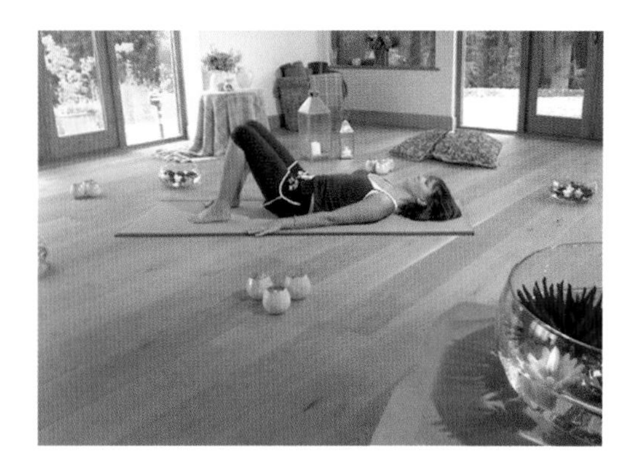

Release the feet down and bring the feet hip width apart, finding a neutral spine, so that you feel that slight natural curve in the lower back. Tilt the pelvis backwards and forwards until you find this middle place.

Engage the core by gathering the stomach muscles in with your pelvic floor zipped up towards the naval, inhaling up into your chest. Exhale, keeping the core engaged.

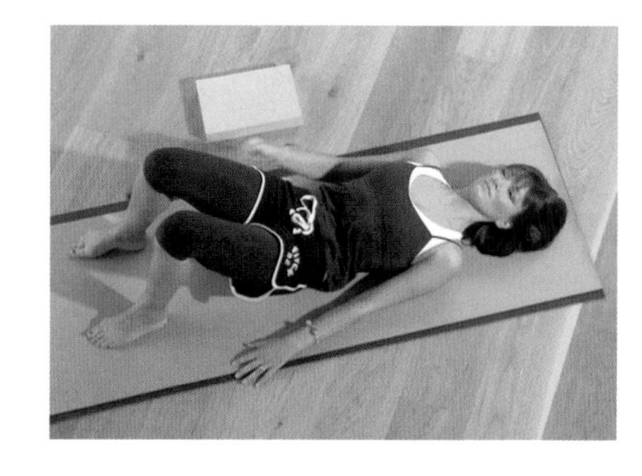

Exhale rolling up and inhale releasing down and repeat four times. Hold the final one at the top giving you one straight line from the knees down to the rib cage, with the lower ribs and core gathered in. Release back down.

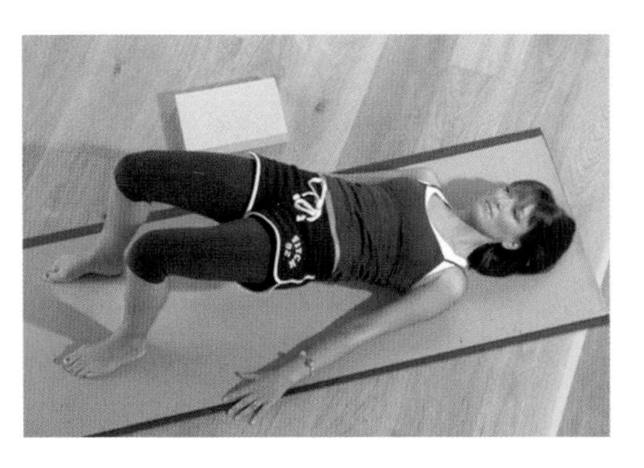

Step 1

Step 2

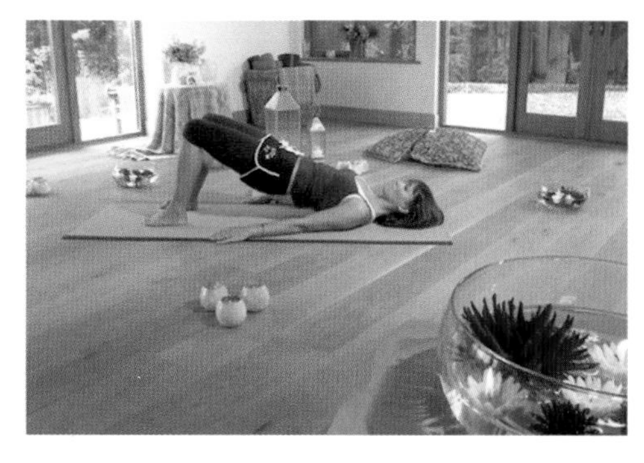

Put a cushion between your knees and as you exhale repeat the above by rolling up, but squeezing the cushion as you roll up and down, exhaling on the way up and inhaling on the way down.

Step 1

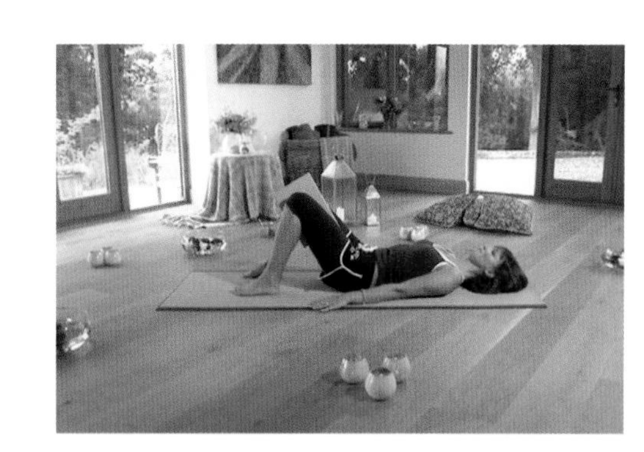

Step 2

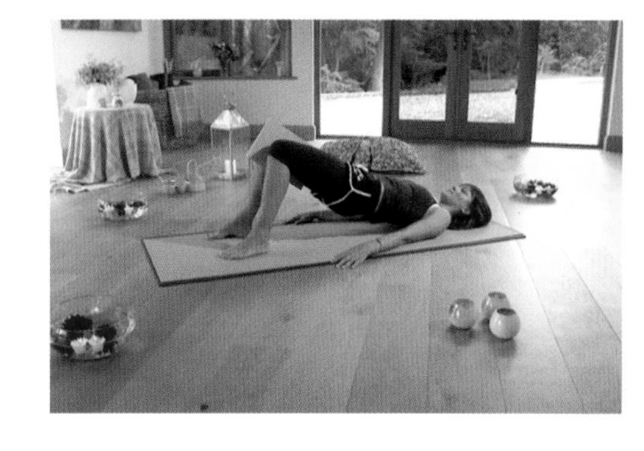

Repeat four times and on the fourth hold the position at the top and bring the arms up behind the head, then roll back down and bring the arms back down beside you.

Step 1

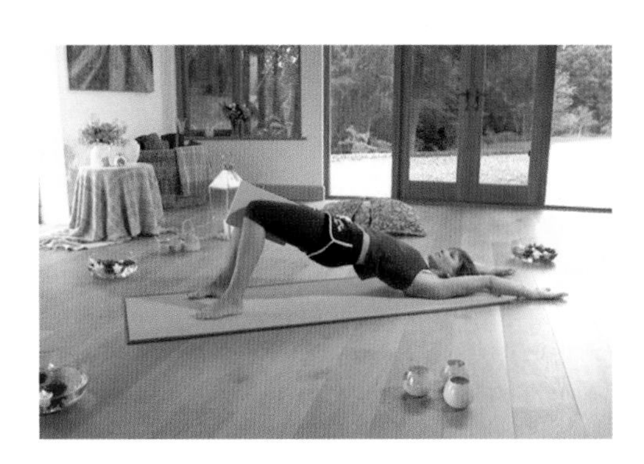

Step 2

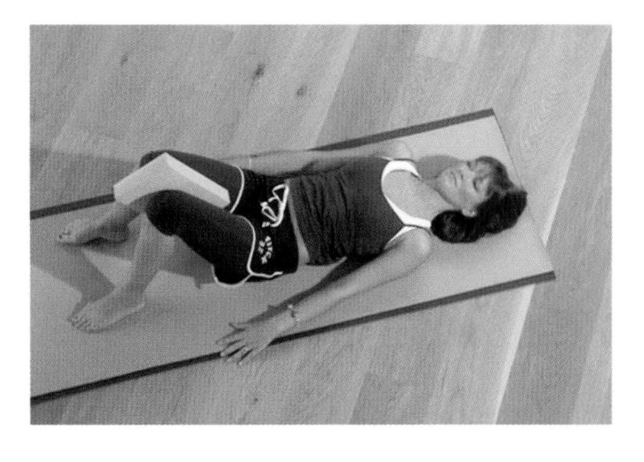

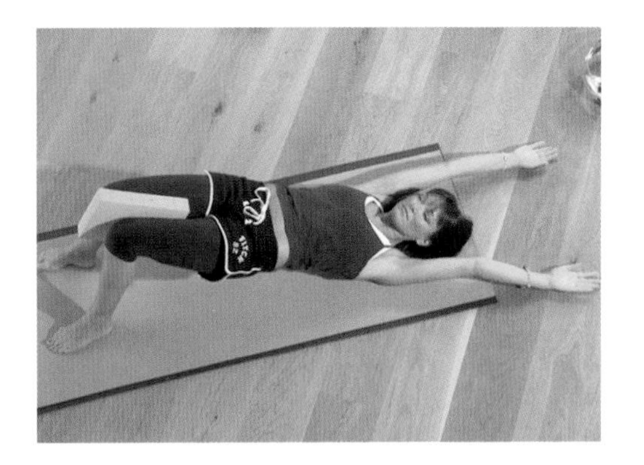

Inhale and roll up again, bring the arms above your head and hold it there, then roll back down, bringing the arms beside you last. Repeat this one more time before taking the cushion away.

Draw your knees into your chest again and gently rock from side to side.

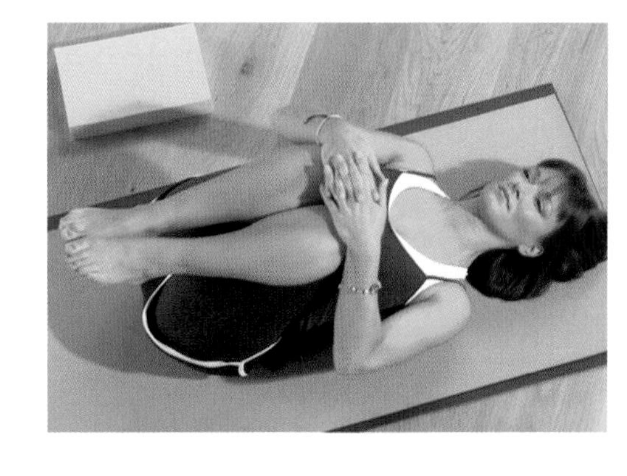

Put your feet on the mat, hip width apart and parallel, and with your pelvis in neutral.

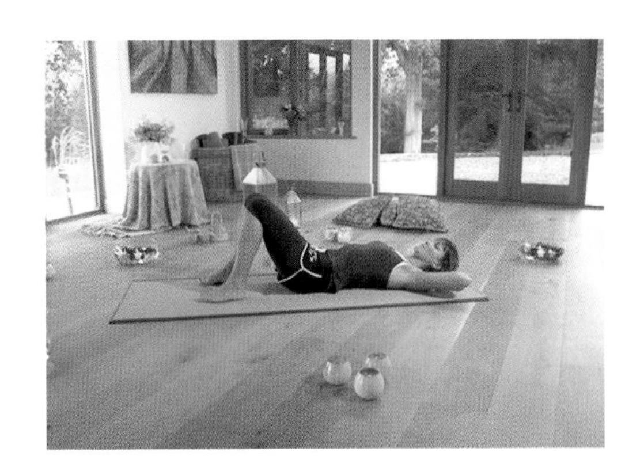

Interlace your hands behind your head, exhale, bringing your head to a hover by using your core to lift yourself up.

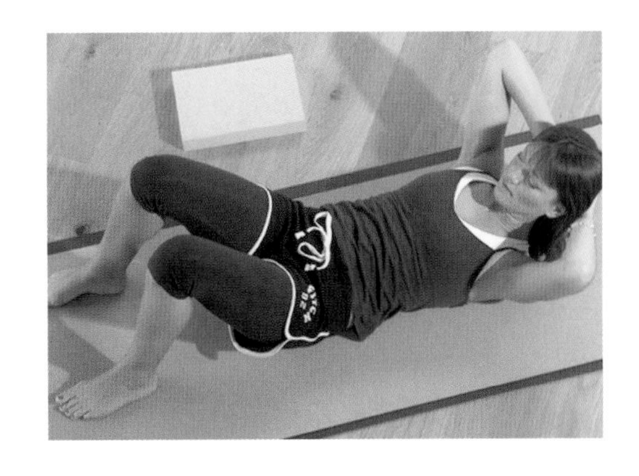

Inhale, then as you exhale move a little higher. Inhale, then exhale curling up as high as you can, holding it there and breathing into it, then releasing down. Repeat this four more times.

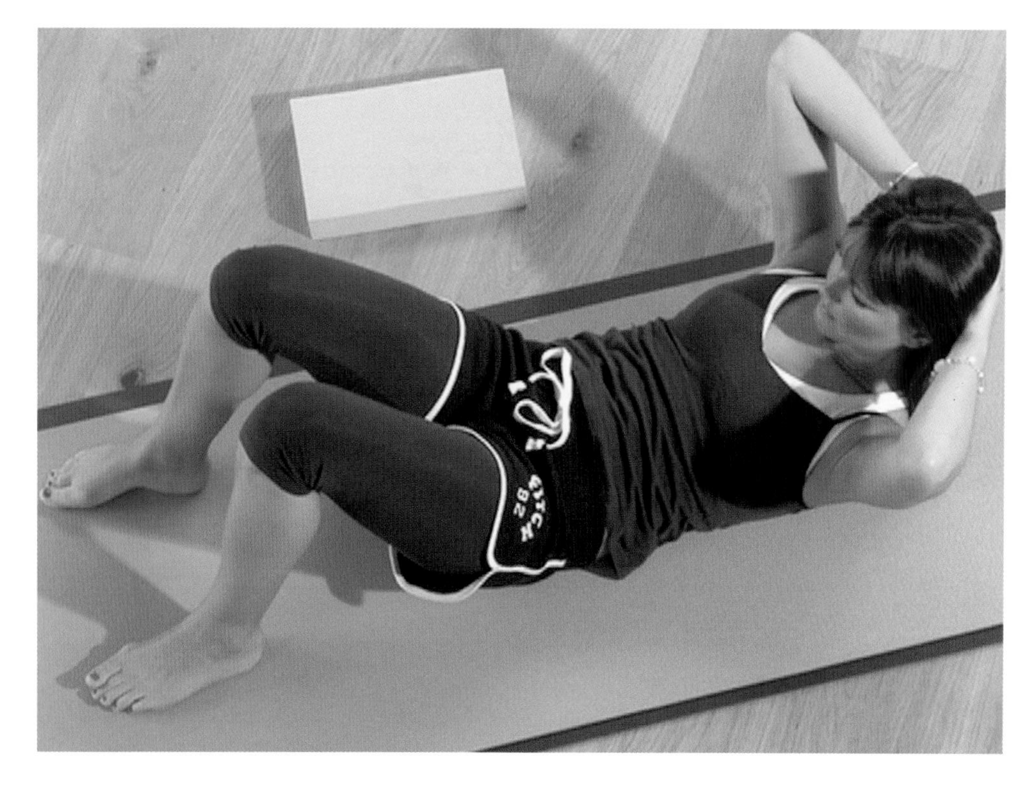

Bring the arms out wide, dropping the knees down to the left.

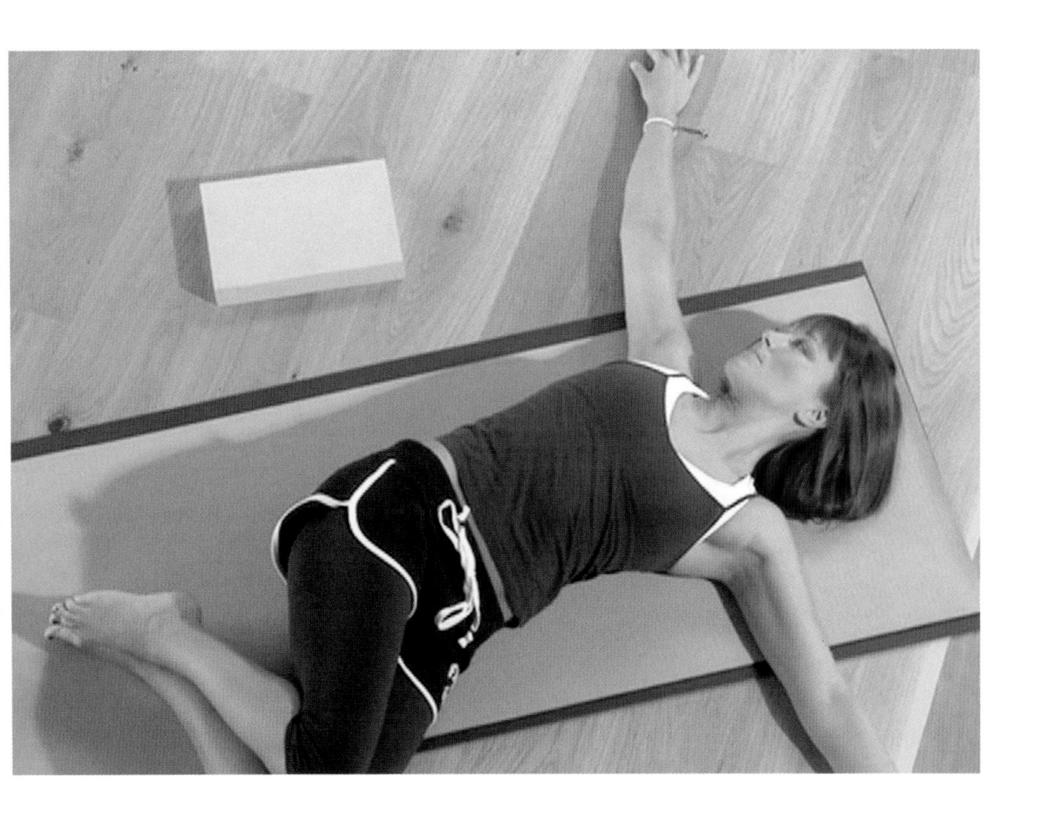

Draw the knees through centre then dropping the knees down to the right. Repeat this one more time.

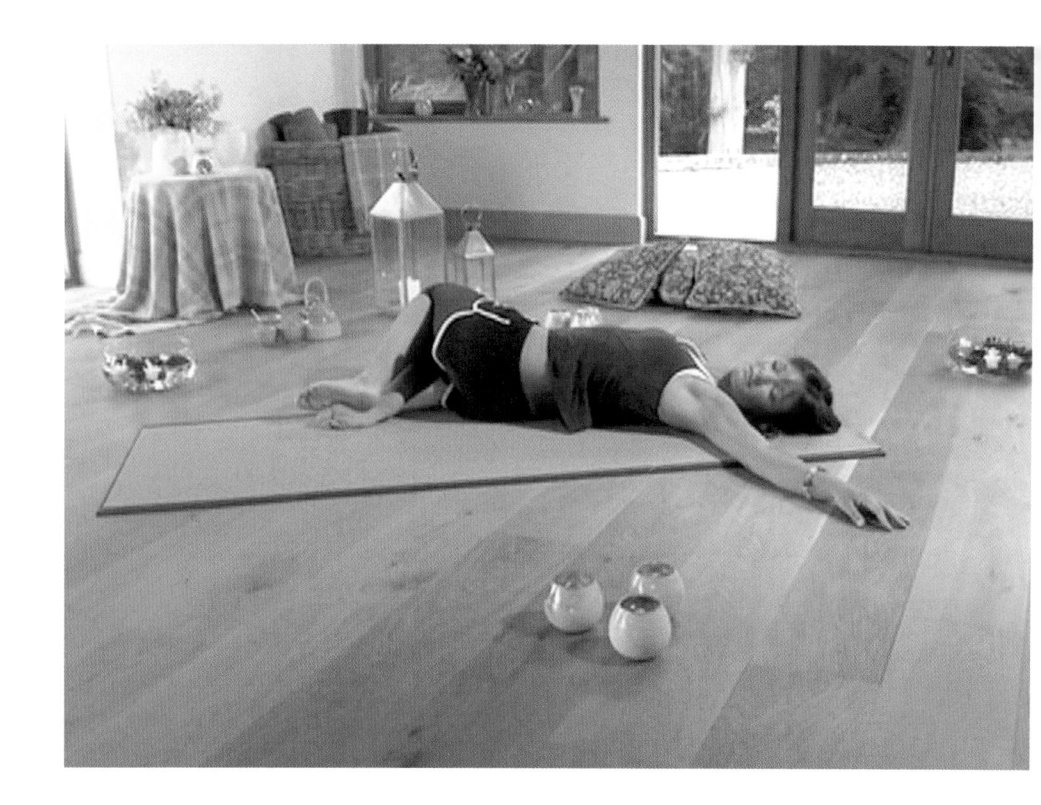

Bring the knees back to centre and bring the feet hip width apart. Bring the right hand behind the head and the left hand and arm hovers off the floor so you're really reaching through your fingers.

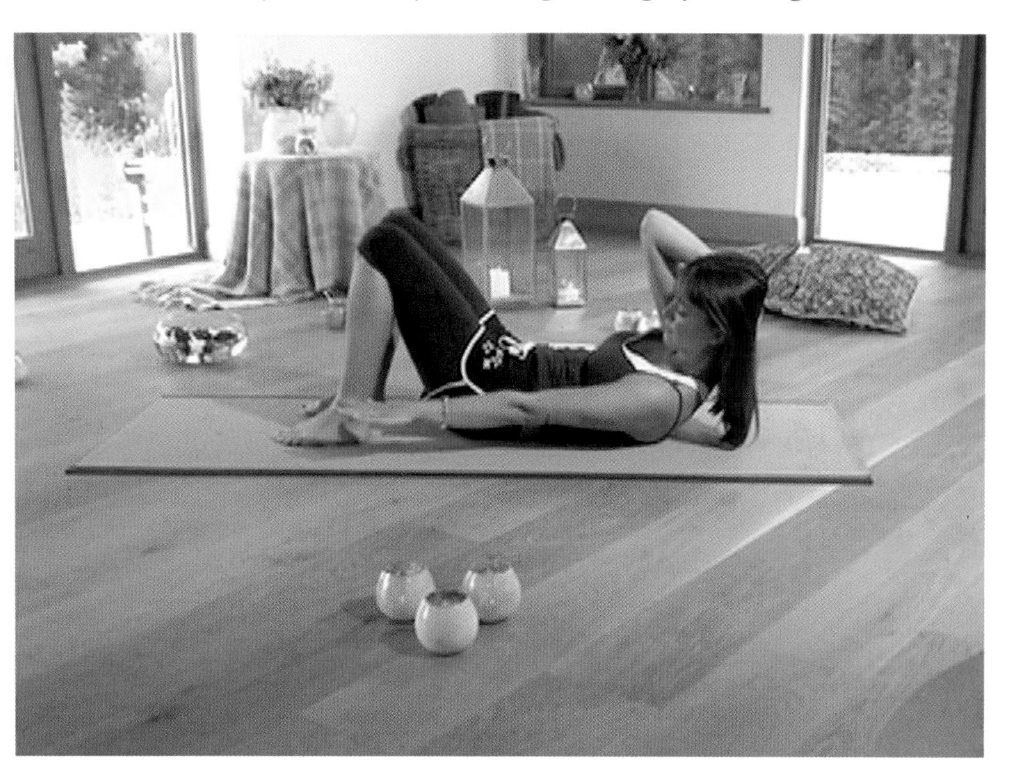

Exhale, and as you do so draw the right elbow towards the left knee, reaching down with the left arm. Inhale down and exhale up. Repeat eight times and then change sides and do the same thing with your left hand behind your head and your right arm hovering off the floor.

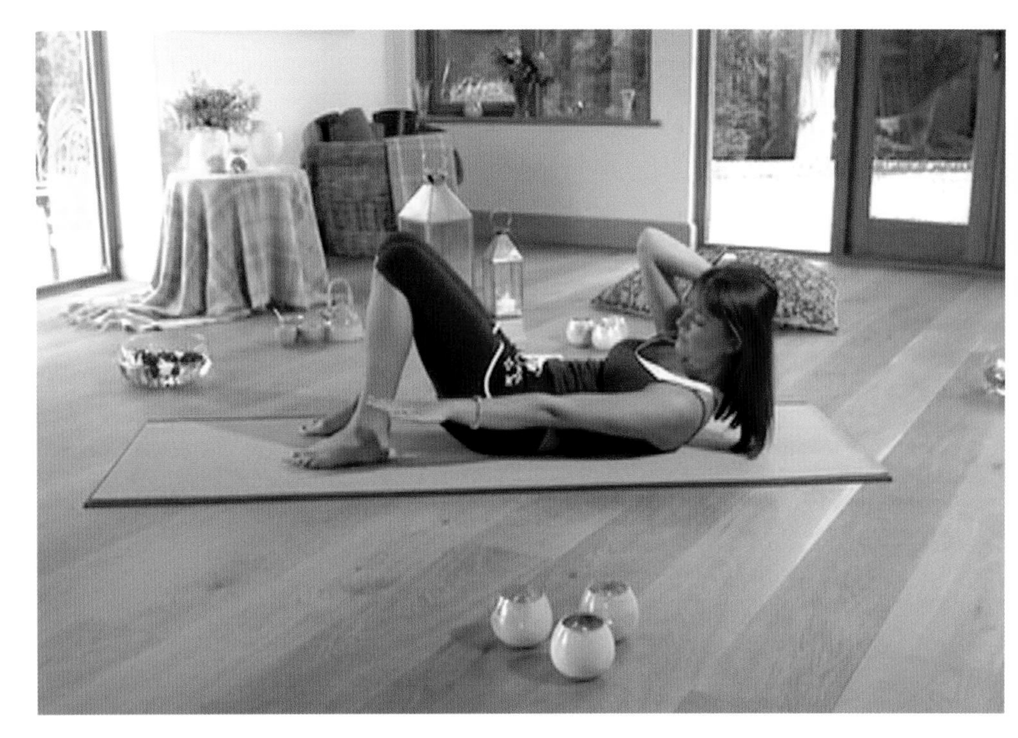

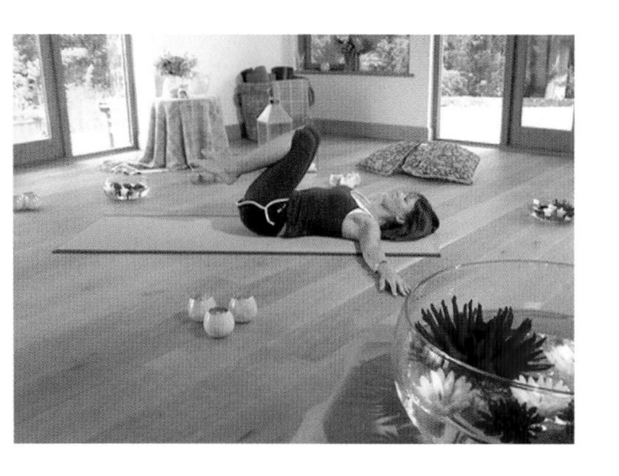

Bring the spine back to neutral and draw your knees in with your feet lifted up off the floor and with your arms out to the side.

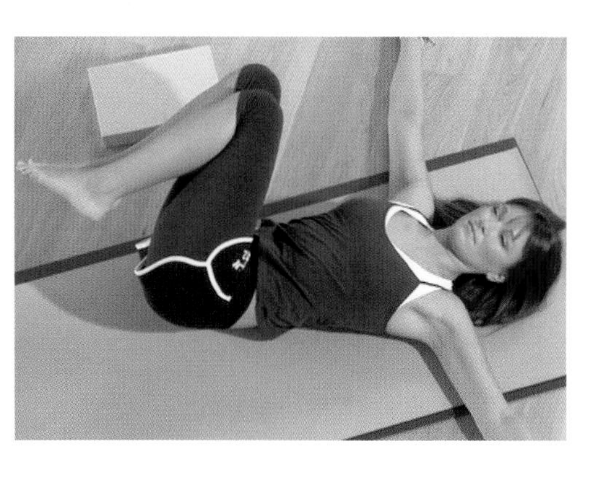

Inhale and draw the knees to the left, exhale to centre, then inhale and draw the knees to the right. Repeat four times.

Do the same as above but this time extend the upper leg as you go from side to side.

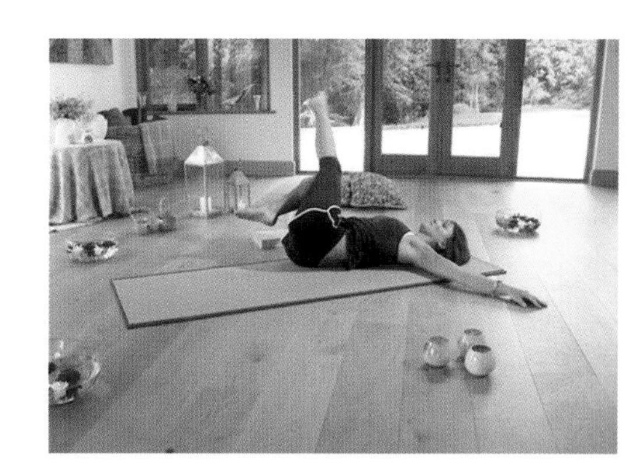

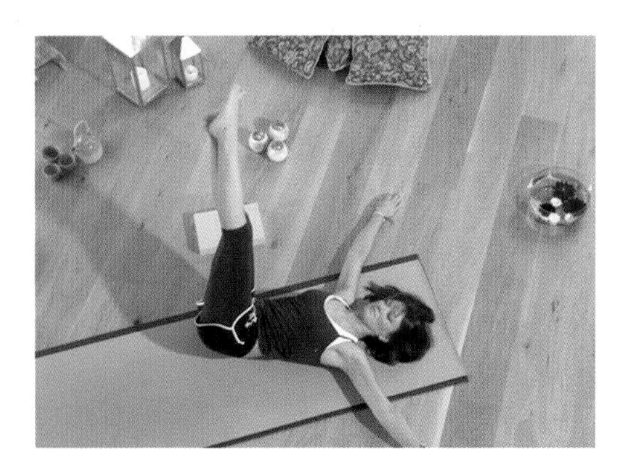

The second option is to extend both legs, which is a little bit more challenging.

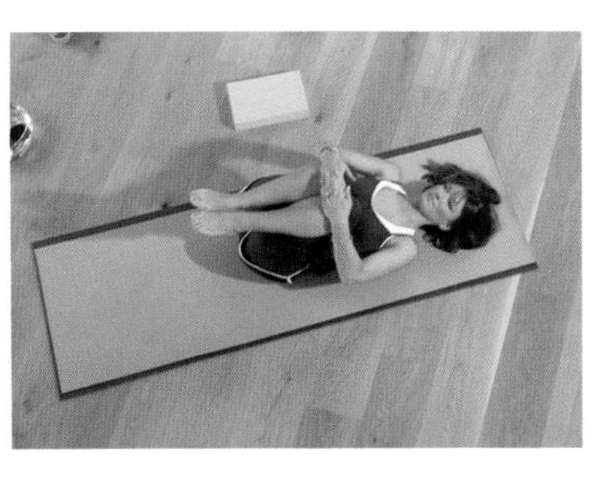

Release and hug your knees into your chest, gently rocking from side to side.

Lie with your lower legs parallel to the floor and knees bent, sinking your lower back down to the floor, core engaged and arms to the side.

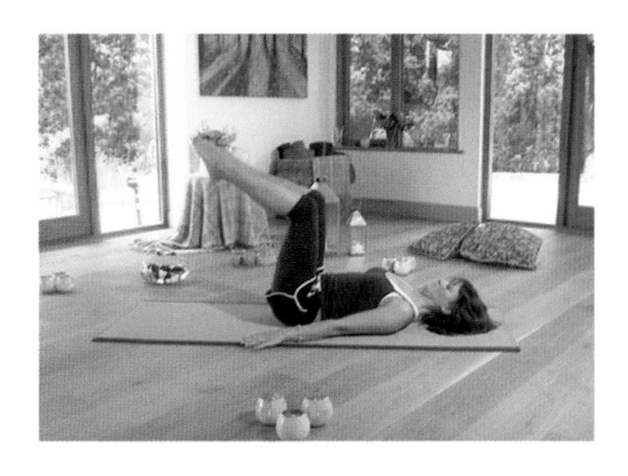

Lower one leg at a time, keeping the leg at a right angle as you lower it to the floor. Inhale up and exhale down. Repeat about 10 times.

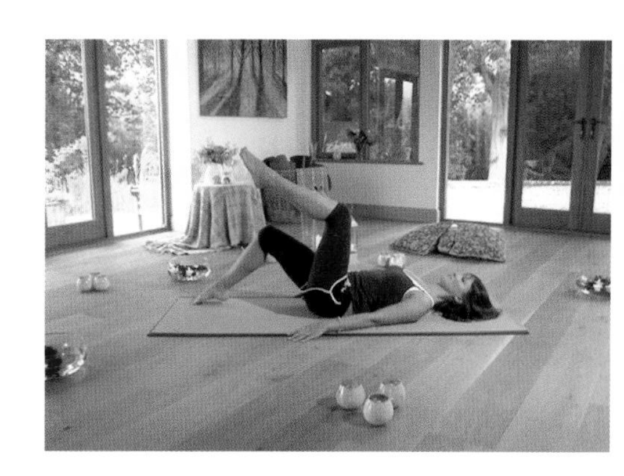

The second stage of this exercise is to lower both legs down together, but it is important here that you make sure your lower back stays pressed down to the floor as you lower the legs. Inhale up, exhale down. Repeat about 10 times.

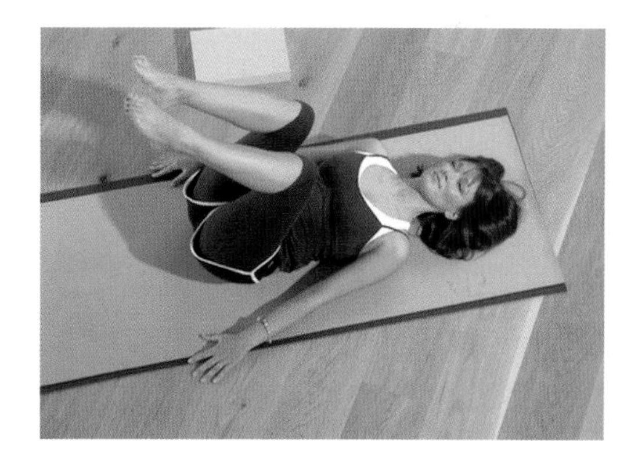

To finish this exercise bring the knees in to the chest and gently rock from side to side.

Bring the right foot onto the left knee, draw the right knee across the body with the right arm out wide, breathing into the stretch. Stretch out the hip and the side of the thigh. Breath into your belly and relax your core. Hold for several seconds and repeat on the other side.

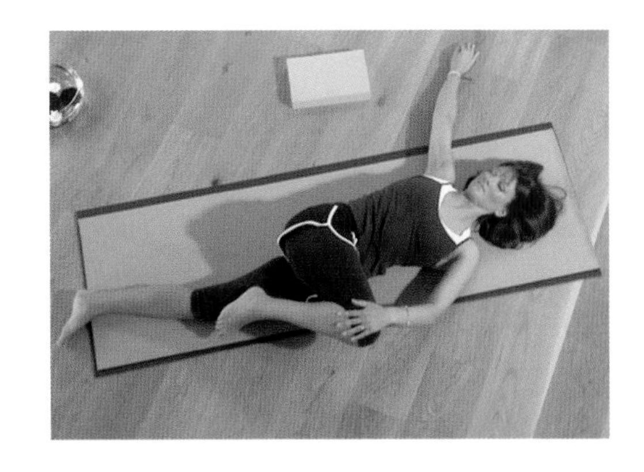

Bring feet back to the centre hip width apart with your arms down beside you with the neutral spine position, hold for several seconds before slowly getting up.

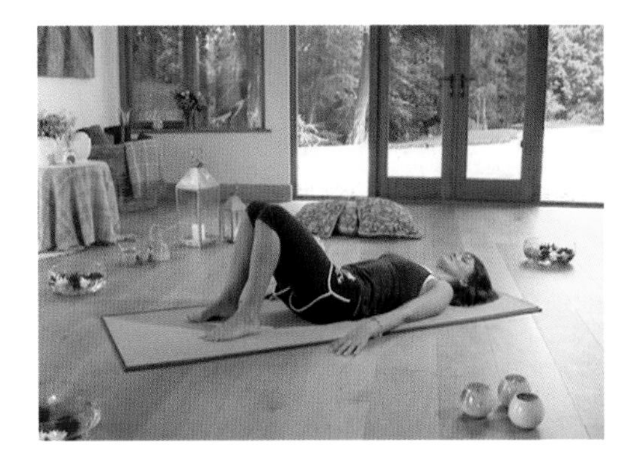

Chapter 3

Toning and Shaping Legs Hips, Arms and Bum

Lie on the floor on your side with your hips and legs one on top of the other - engage the core with your pelvic floor zipped up into the naval and breathing right up into the chest.

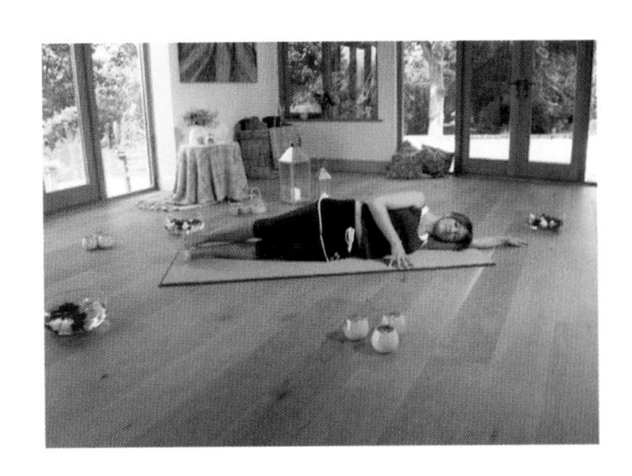

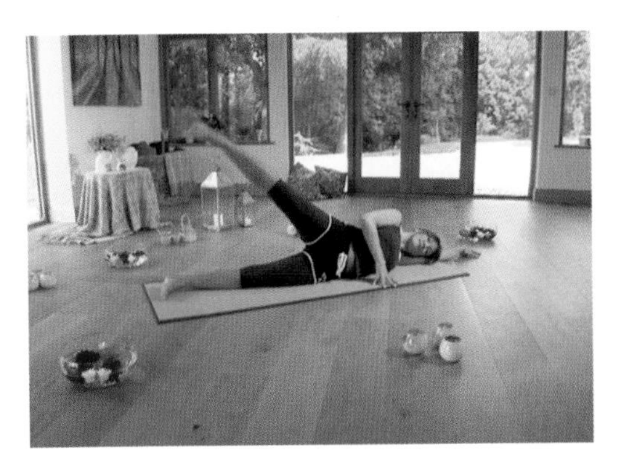

Inhale to prepare and then as you exhale lift the top leg up a little and begin to circle the top leg around. Start by doing small circles and then gradually increase the size of the circles, breathing into each one, keeping a nice flowing movement. Repeat about 20 times and then circle the leg in the opposite direction.

Release the leg back parallel with the bottom leg, then draw the leg forward as far as you can and then backwards as far as you can, keeping your balance. Repeat about 10 times then release the leg back to lie on top of the bottom one.

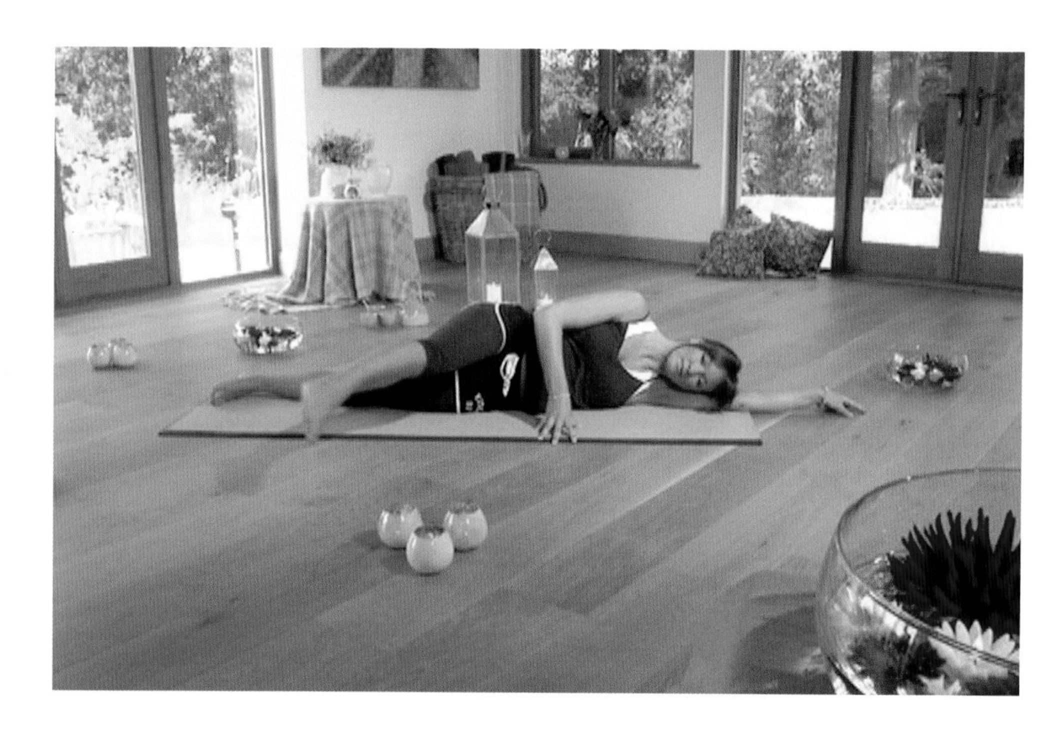

Stay lying on the same side and either slide the knee forward or, if you can, pick the foot up and draw it in front of the bottom leg and hold onto the ankle. Lift the bottom leg up as high as you can, squeezing the inner thigh as you lift it up. Inhale down and exhale as you lift the leg up. Repeat about 20 times.

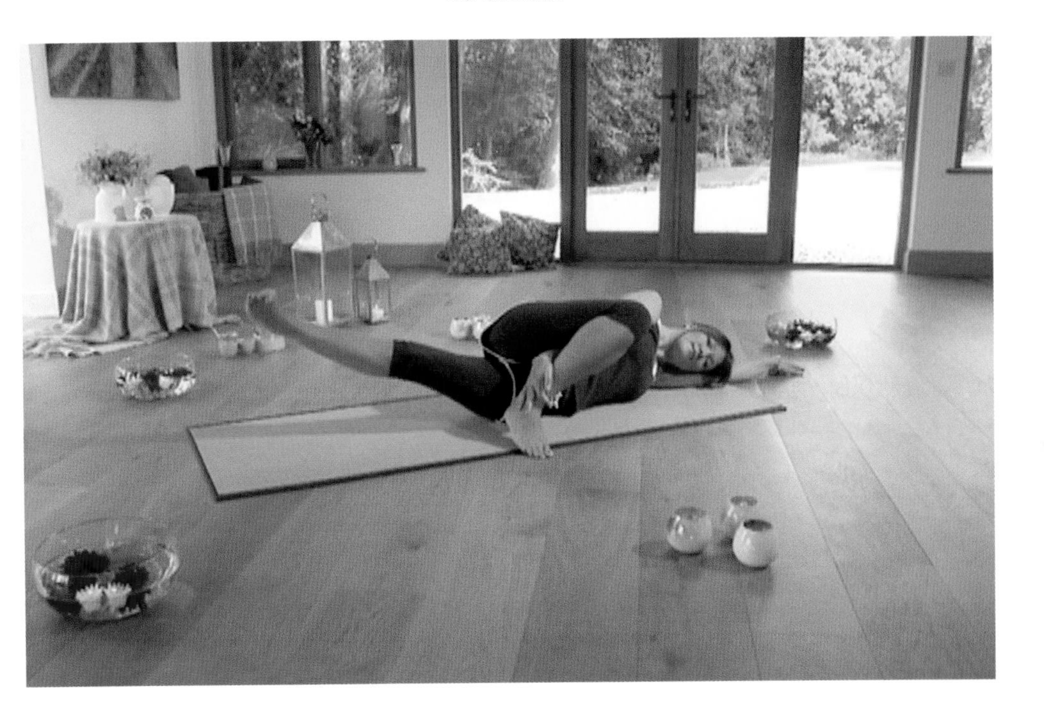

Hold the leg in the high position and then pulse the raised leg up and down 20 times.

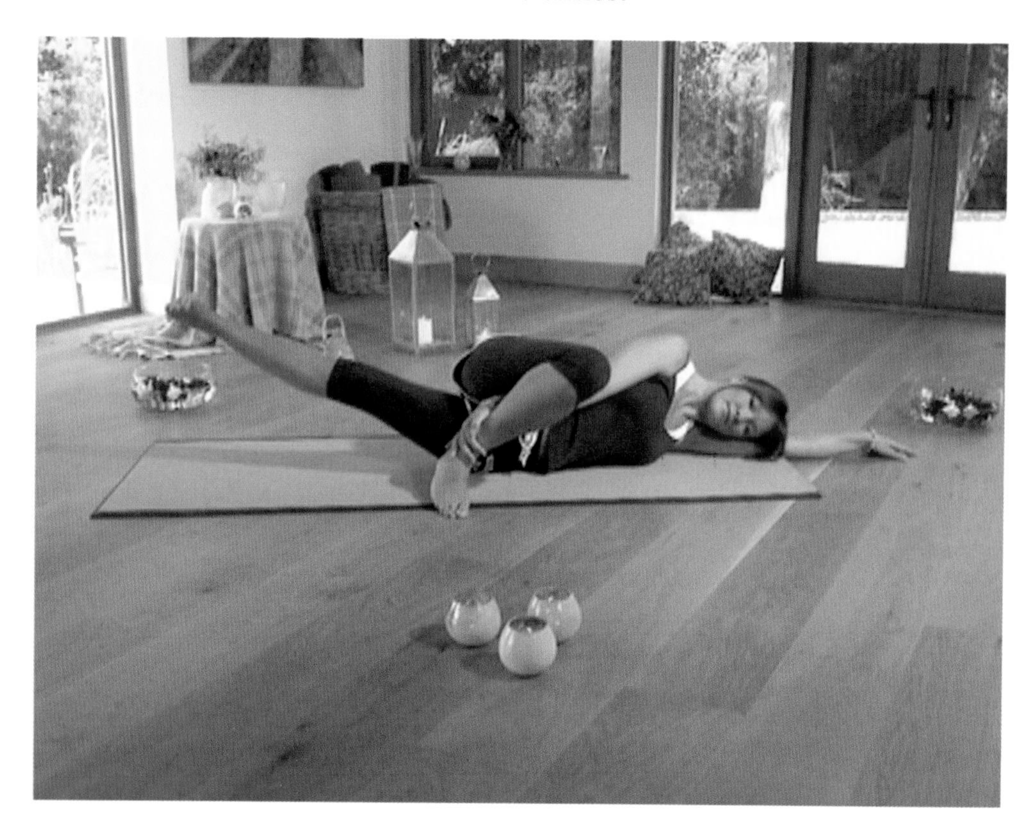

Draw the knees on top of each other and stretch over to the side and hold for several seconds.

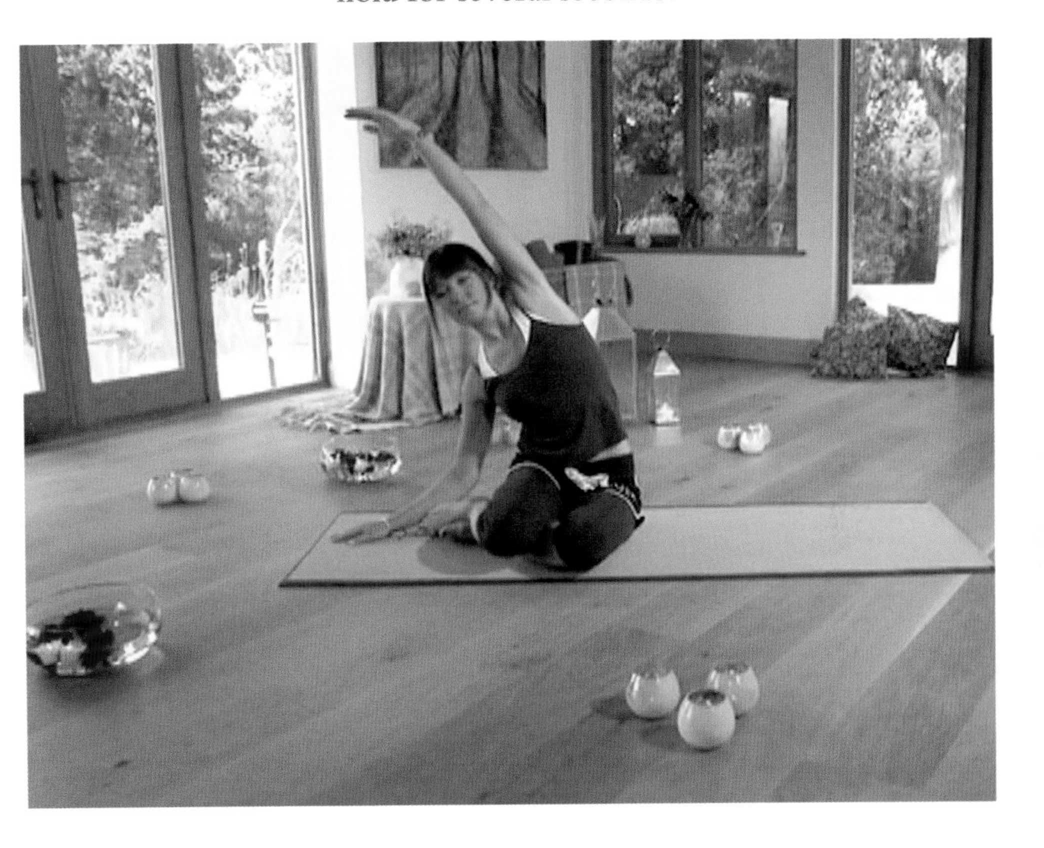

Bring the top leg in front, lifting the hip up and stretching the top arm up and over, engage the core and put some pressure into the front foot. Then release back down and repeat the exercise four times.

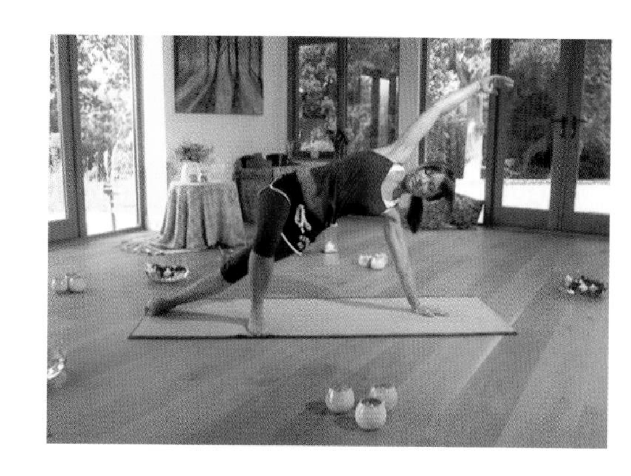

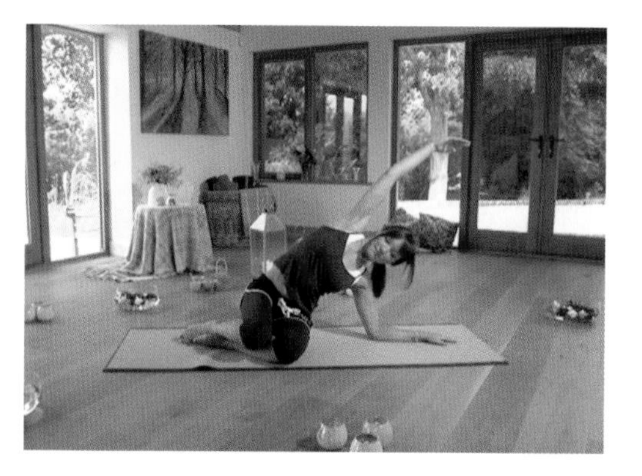

Draw the knees on top of each other and stretch over to the side and hold for several seconds. Repeat the stretch on the other side.

Repeat all of the above exercises lying on your other side.

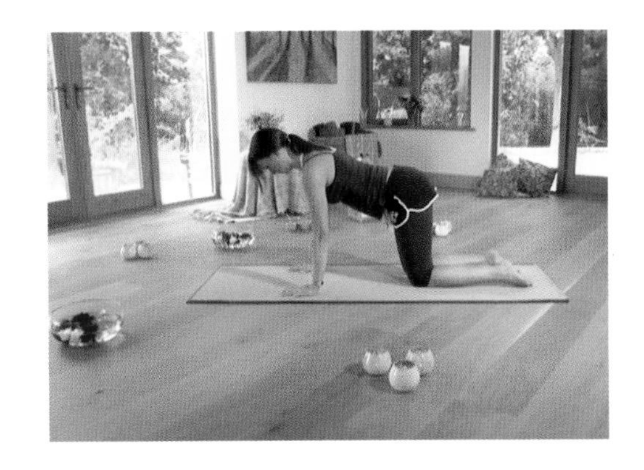

Come onto your hands and knees with your hands underneath your shoulders and knees underneath the hips, finding neutral spine by tilting the pelvis backwards and forwards until you find that neutral position.

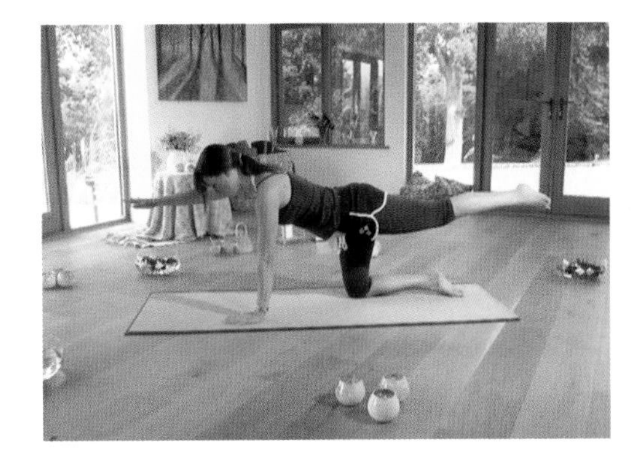

Gather in your core and raise your left leg back, keeping the hips directly in line and then raise the right arm forward coming into a balance and working the whole of the body. Keep the neck in line with the spine by tucking your chin slightly into your neck. Hold for several seconds and release back down. Repeat raising your right leg back and left arm forward.

On your hands and knees, draw your right leg in towards your forehead as it curls down to meet the knee, rounding the back. Exhale and lift the head slowly back up as the right leg goes back, squeezing the bum, then pulsing the leg up and down for 10 repetitions.

Step 1

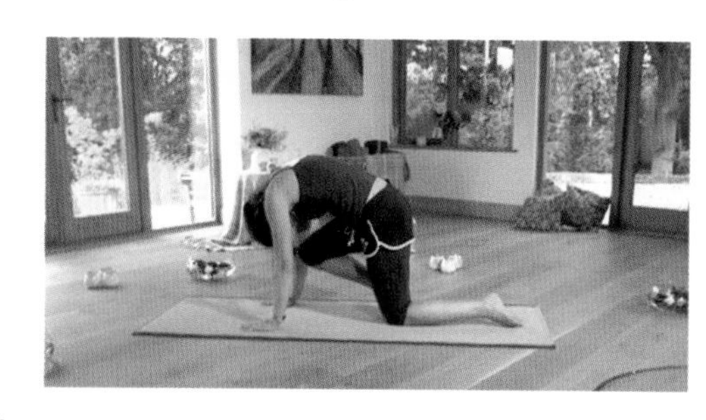

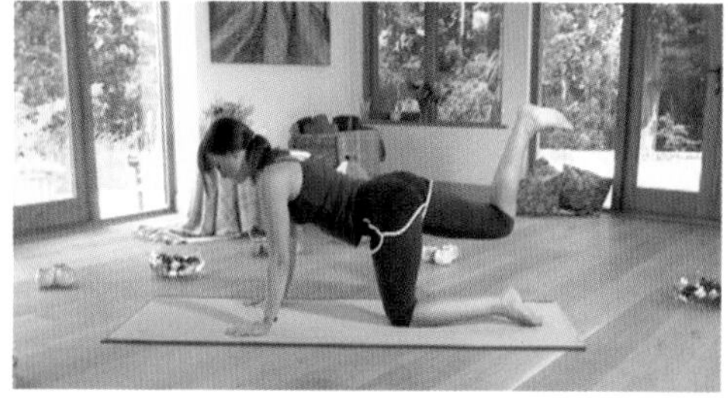

Step 2

Inhale and bring your knee back towards your forehead and repeat the pulsing once your leg is back. Repeat twice more with your right leg and then repeat the exercise with your left leg.

Sit back onto your heels with your hands stretched out in front of you, resting down into 'child's pose', stretched forward and breathing into the belly. Hold for several seconds.

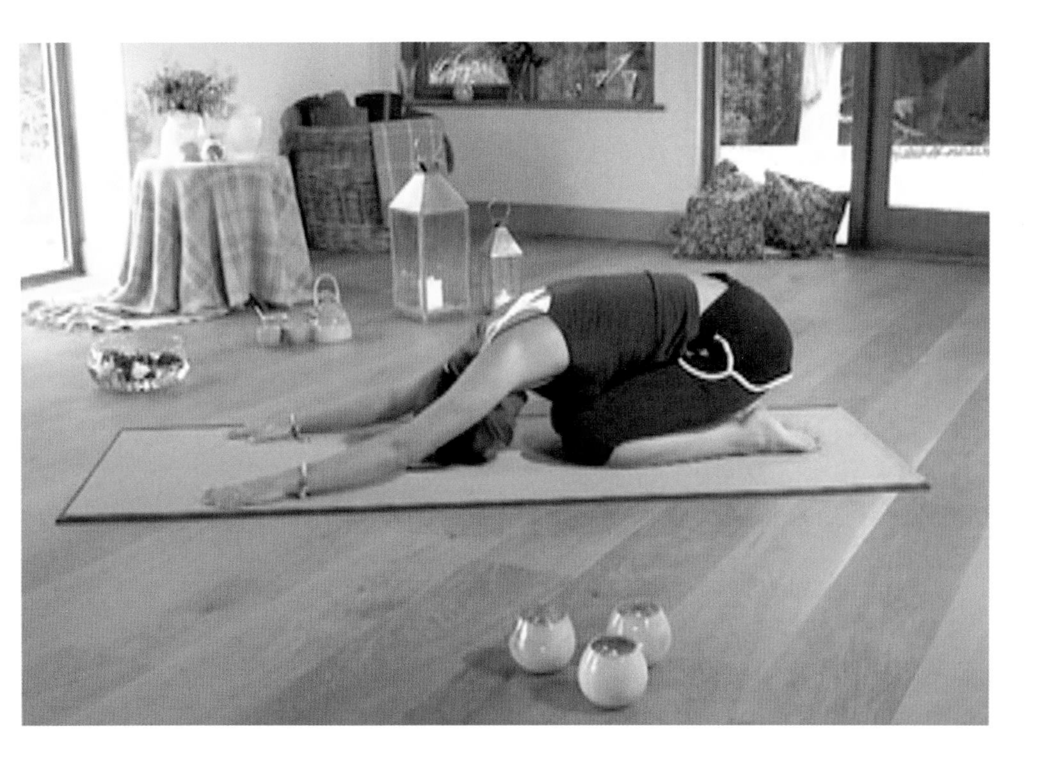

Come back up onto your hands and knees and push up into a 'cat stretch', stretching the spine up towards the ceiling, rounding the back. Then release through centre and stretch out the front of the body. Repeat 3 more times.

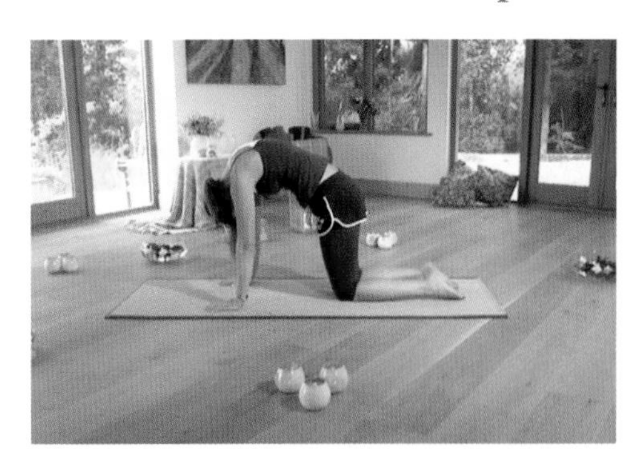

Step 1

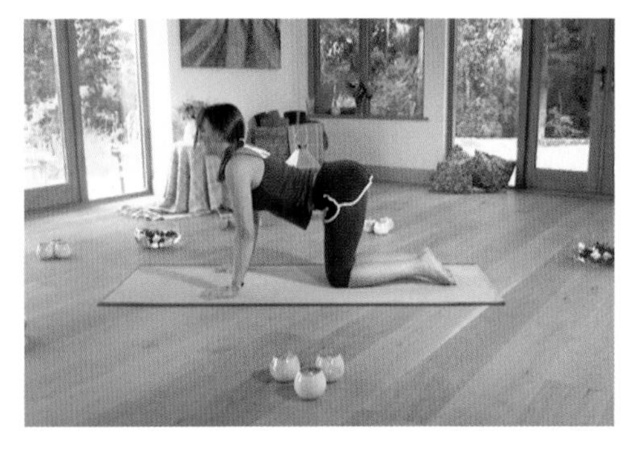

Step 2

Go back to the centre on your hands and knees, then tuck your toes under and push up on your arms keeping your elbows bent and knees bent to begin with, stretch your tailbone as high as you can, straightening your knees and elbows at the same time, known as 'downward facing dog'.

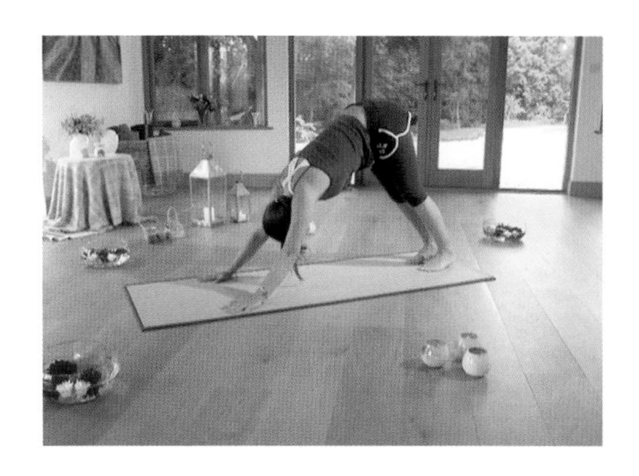

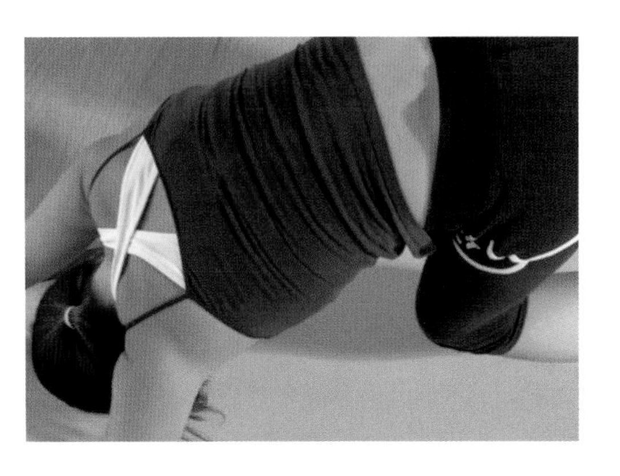

If this stretch gets too much at any time just release back down.

Stretch out the legs one at a time by bending one knee and then the other, making sure that the core is engaged and keeping the tailbone lifted high.

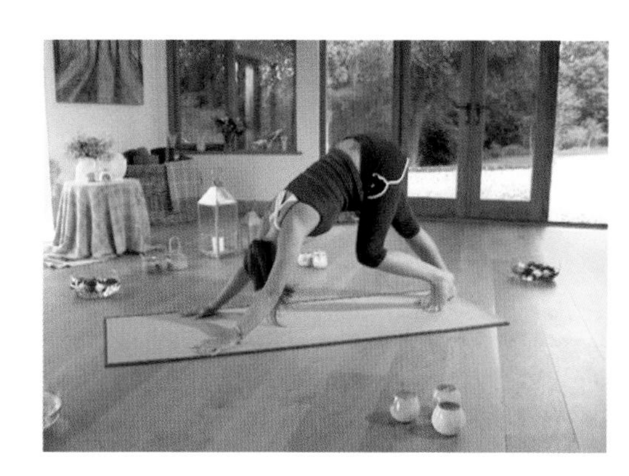

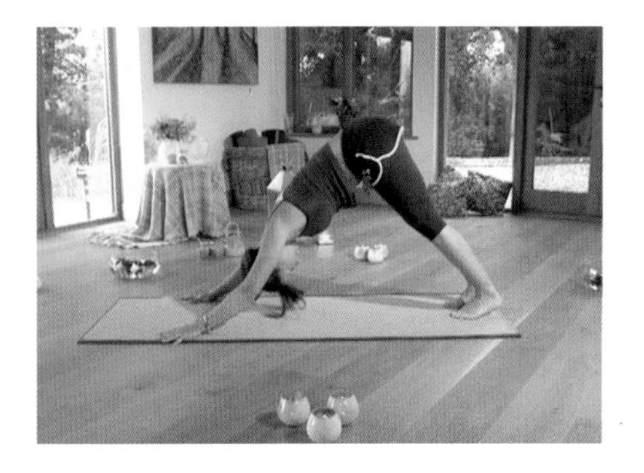

Push both heels down towards the floor and pulling up on the front of the thighs and lifting the kneecaps upwards, engaging with the quadriceps muscles and lifting the tailbone high. Hold for several seconds.

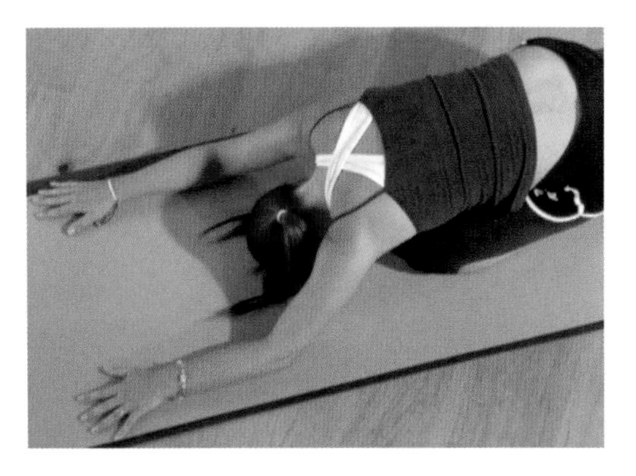

Release back down onto all fours and then lean back on the heels and relax, taking a few deep breaths, relaxing the core muscles by breathing into the belly.

Come back up onto your hands and knees and tucking the toes under, lifting again into 'downward facing dog' as above. Hold for several seconds, then release back down and sit back on your heels, relaxing.

Walk your hands around to one side until you feel a stretch on the side of one arm and let the stomach muscles relax. Walk the hands through centre and then round to the other side, stretching the other arm, breathing deeply all the time.

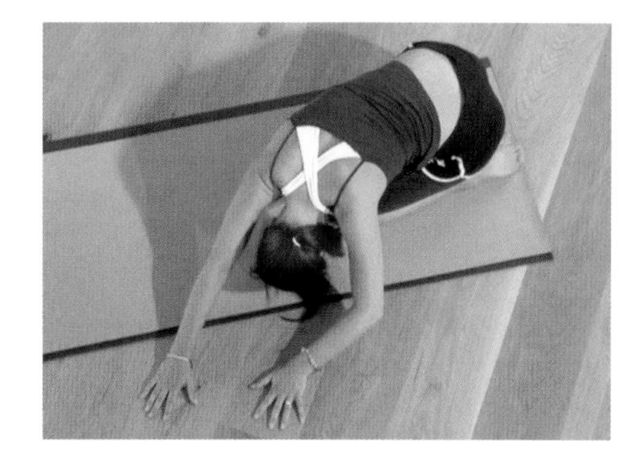

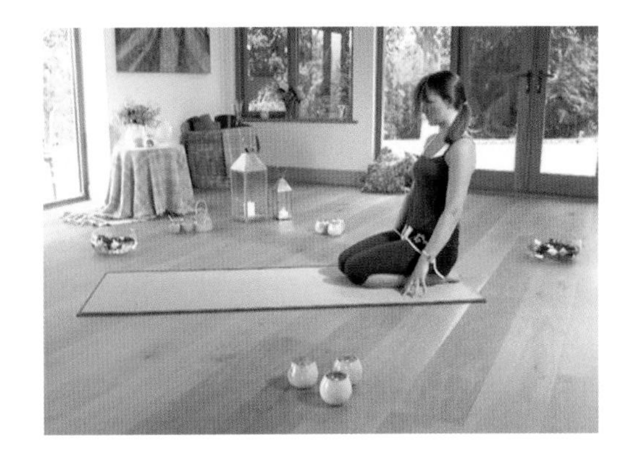

Release back to centre stretching the arms back out in front and then slowly uncurl so you're sitting back on your heels.

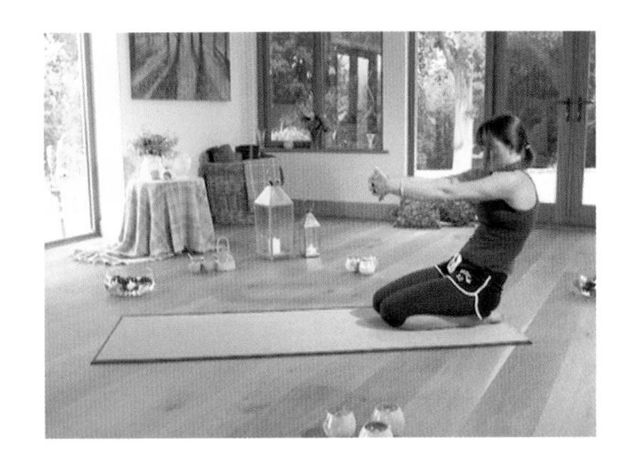

Interlace your hands in front of you and sink back, stretching out the upper back and hold for several seconds.

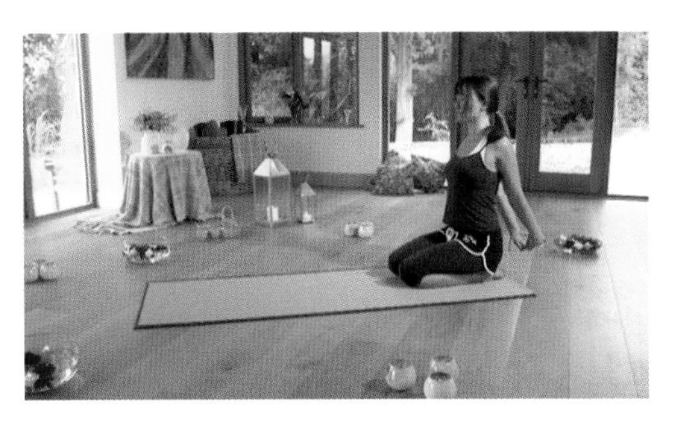

Interlace the hands behind the back, opening the chest and stretching out the shoulders and chest. Breath into the belly with the core relaxed.

Stretch out the wrists by putting your hands on the mat with your fingers facing back towards your feet. Stretch out the wrists by flexing one hand back and then the other one.

Step 1

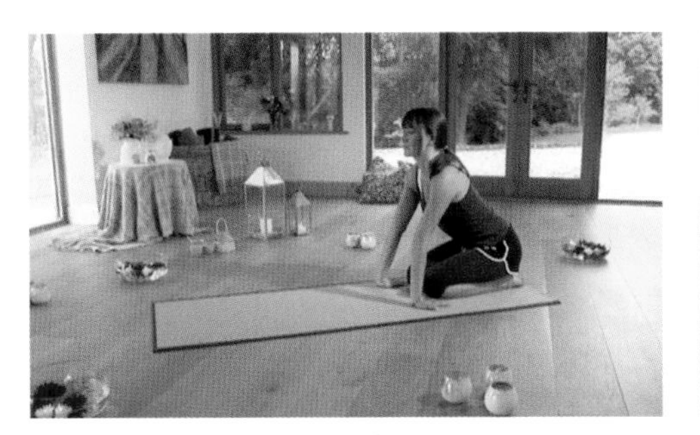

Step 2

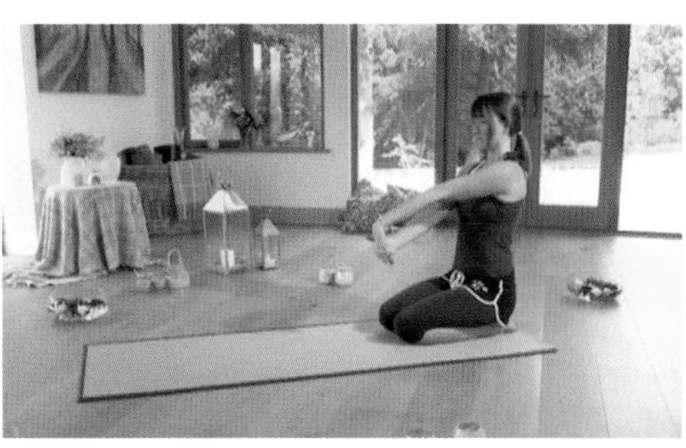

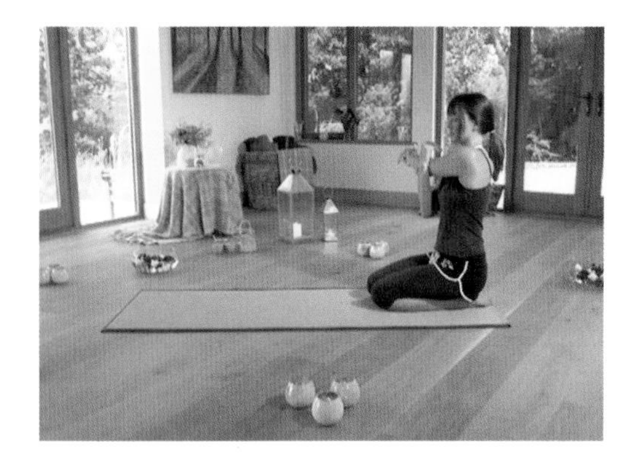

Bring one arm across the body, easing it across with the other and then repeat with the other arm.

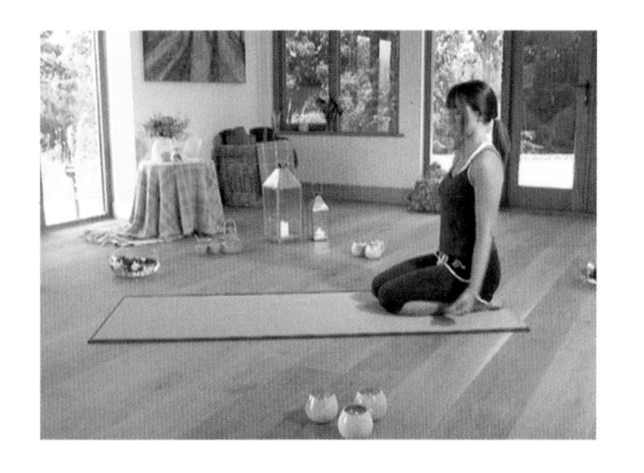

Release the arms down and loosen the shoulders by rolling them back a few times.

Chapter 4

Balancing Postures for Alignment

Lie on the mat in 'child's pose' with your arms down beside you, head relaxed and then stretch out your arms.

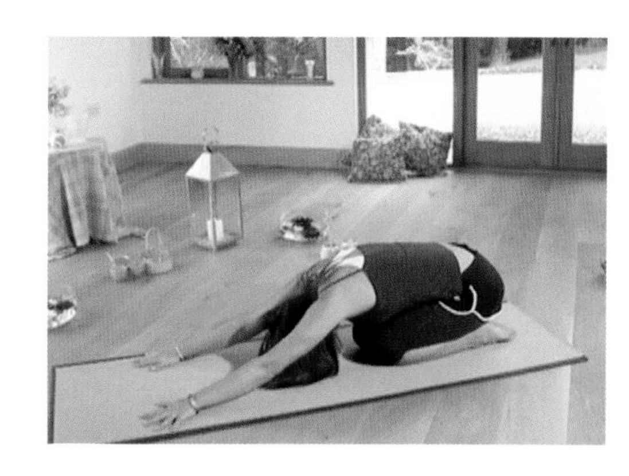

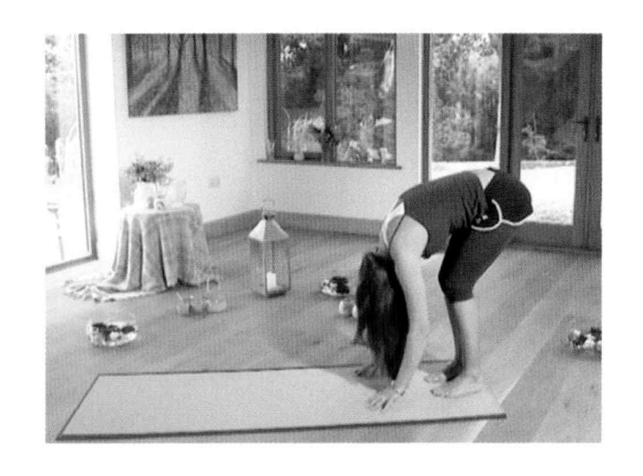

Slowly uncurl and tucking your toes under, lift your tailbone high and relaxing the upper body down come into a forward fold, letting the head relax.

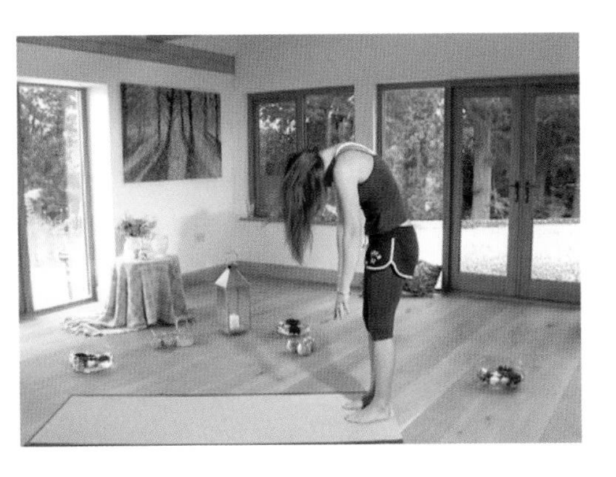

Gather your navel in and begin to uncurl the spine vertebra by vertebra.

Inhale raising the arms up and bring the palms together, coming up onto the toes and stretching high, then release the arms back down by your side. Repeat the stretch.

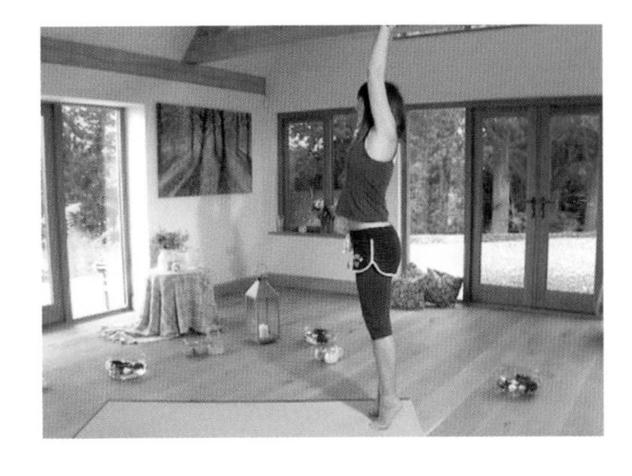

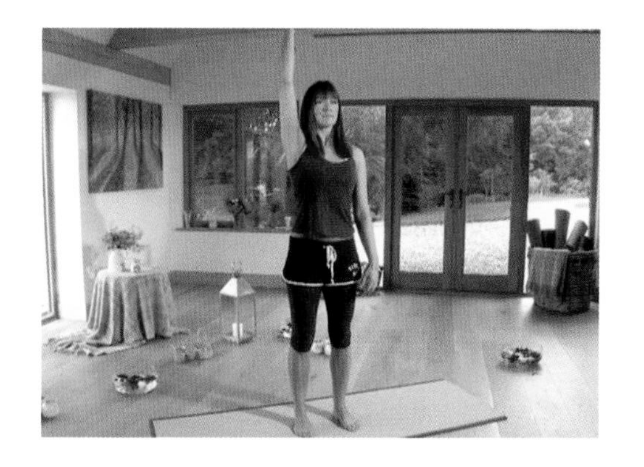

Stand on the mat with feet hip width apart and feet parallel. Bring the pelvis into neutral spine and lift and lengthen through the spine and neck, standing really tall.

Bring your shoulders back and down so they are nice and open, then roll your shoulders backwards a few times to get them in this position.

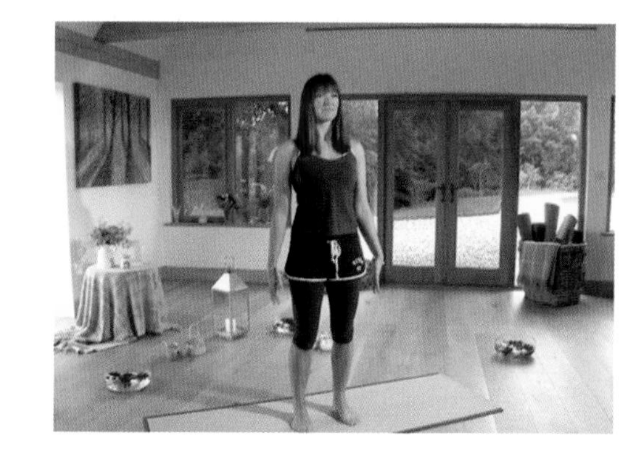

Put your hands onto your hips. Known as 'tree pose', place one foot onto your ankle, lifting it a little higher if you feel balanced. It can go just below the knee, above the knee or even right up onto the inner thigh. Palms together. Keep the hips in line and core lightly engaged.

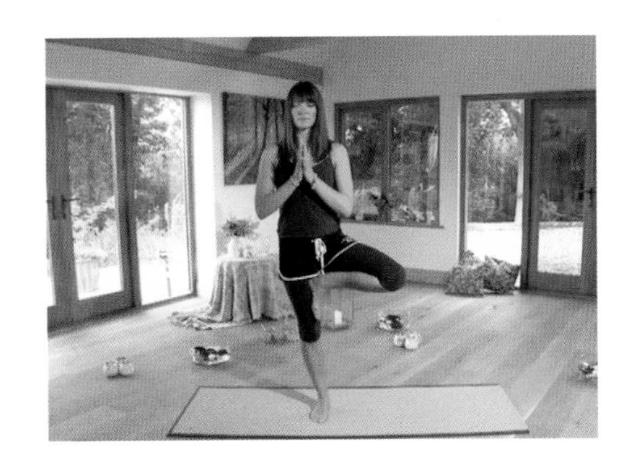

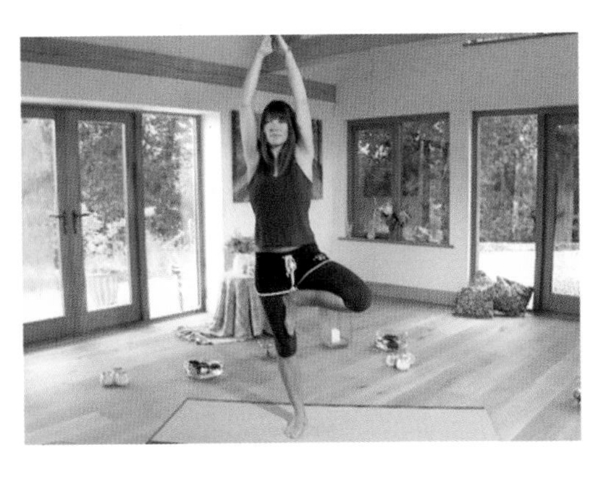

Lift your hands above your head with your palms together and stretching high. Repeat with the other leg.

Put the weight on one leg and lift the other knee up. Bring the arms out wide, flexing the hands back, stretching through the wrists. Relax the tops of your shoulders and begin to circle the lifted knee around in flowing circles, working the hip joint. Circle the knee the other way.

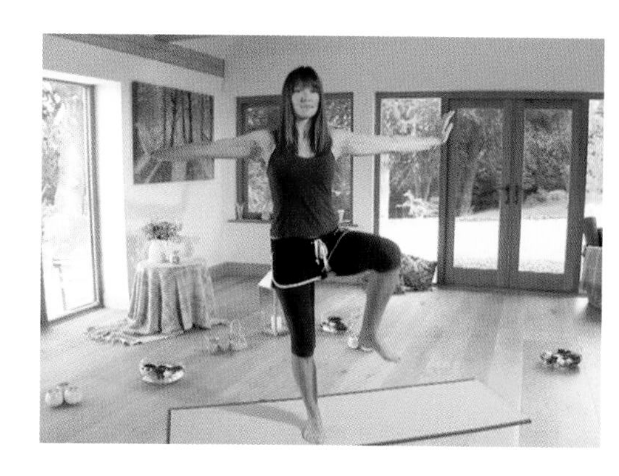

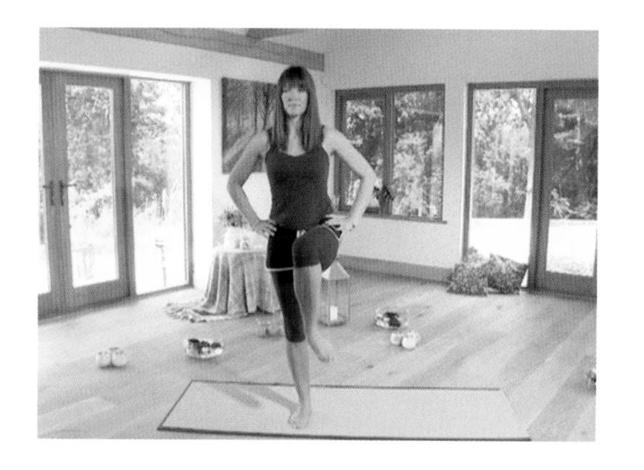

Put your hands back on hips and circle your ankle one way and then the other. Then release and give your leg a shake out. Repeat the exercise with the other knee raised.

Put your weight onto one leg, picking up the other one and holding onto it from the inside of the foot. Tuck your tailbone under and push your hips forward so that you feel the stretch on the thigh. Keeping the leg on the floor strong and grounded, start to kick the other foot back into the hand. If you feel balanced you can raise the front arm up, putting your thumb and first finger together. Repeat on the other leg.

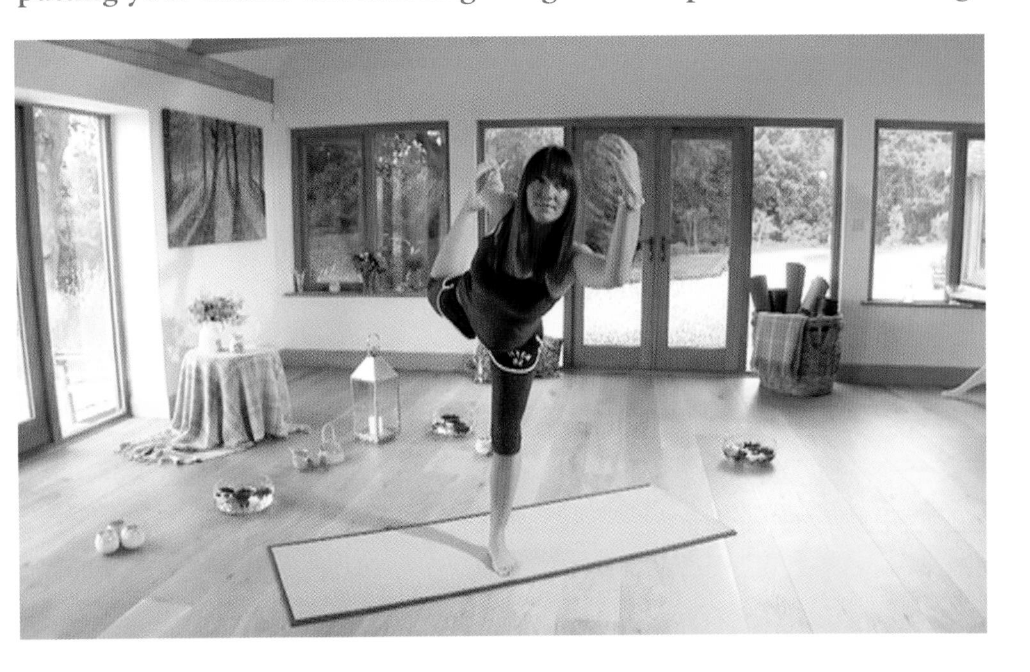

Stand on the mat with your feet hip width apart, bring one leg forward and put your hands on your hips. Moving onto the toes of the back leg, engage the core and slowly lift the back leg up, keeping your hips in line and neck in line with your spine. If you feel balanced, you can stretch your arms forward; a pose known as 'warrior three'. Repeat on the other leg

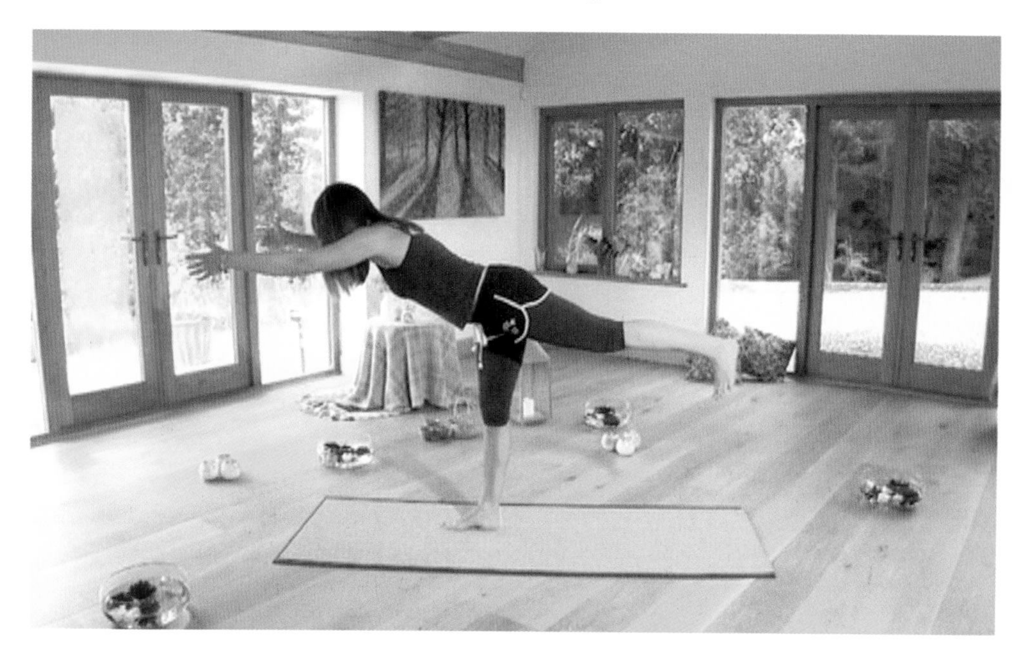

Stand with one foot back, engage the thighs, and put hands on hips. Interlace your hands behind your back, opening the chest. Fold forward with a straight back and slowly bring your hands up towards the ceiling. Release your hands, uncurl slowly bringing your feet back together and repeat on the other leg.

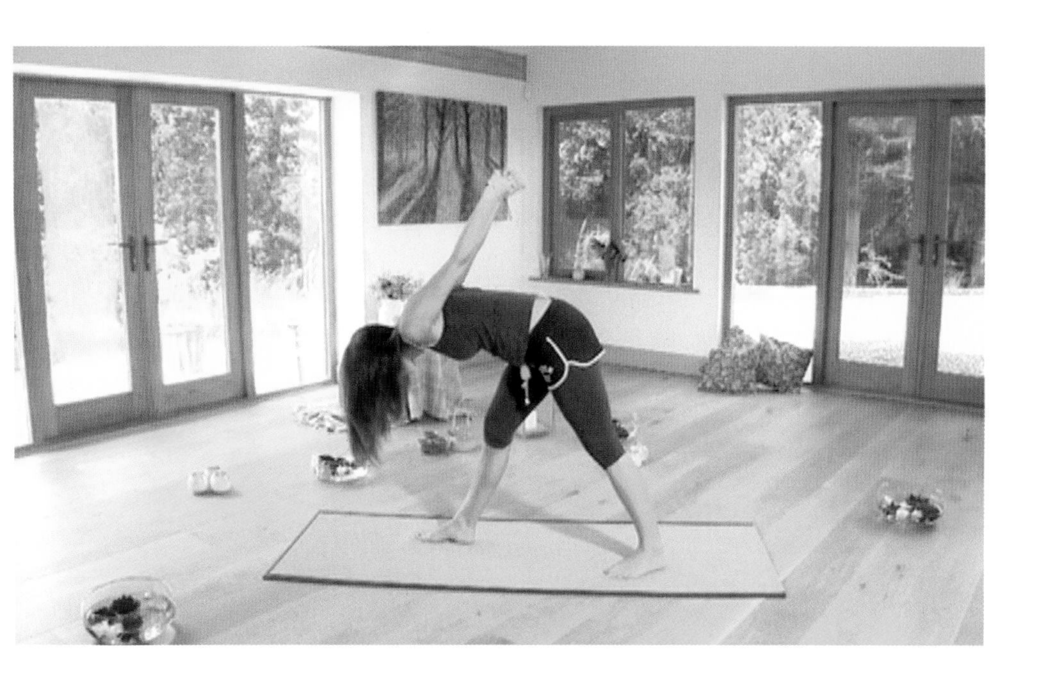

Stand with feet a bit wider than the hips. Drop down into a squat position and draw the elbows in front of the knees, using the arms to push the knees out wide. Bring the palms of the hands together, stretching out the lower back. Lift and open the chest here.

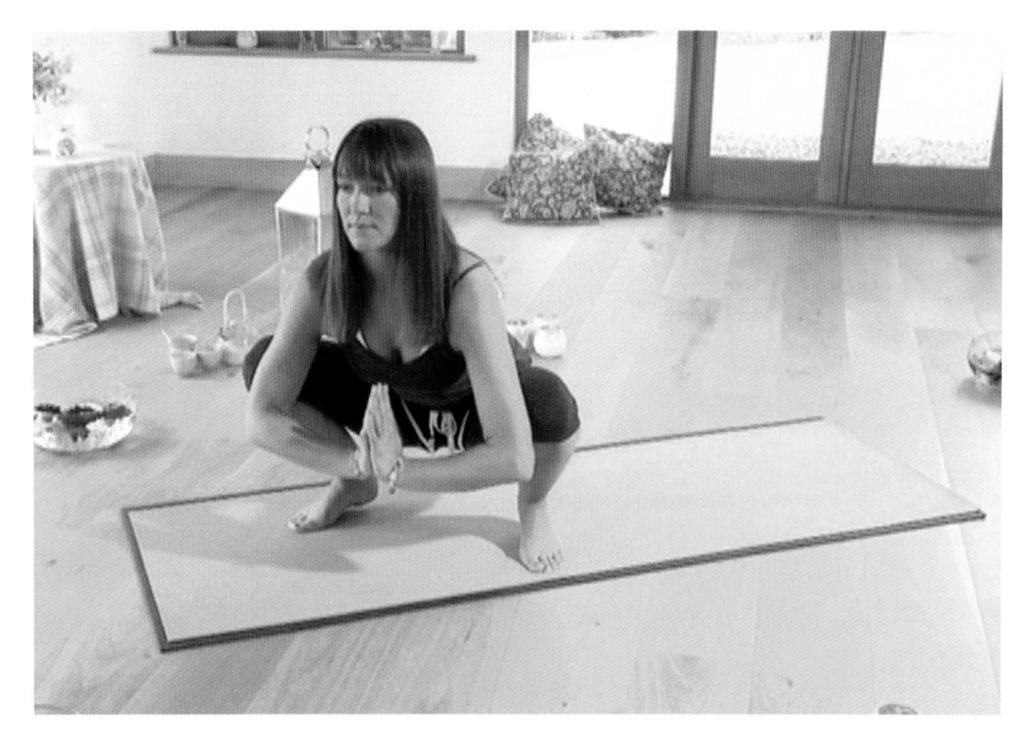

From the previous position interlace the hands, with index finger pointing forwards and stretch the arms out forwards. Finding your balance, come up onto your toes, lifting the heels high. Hold for a few seconds then release back down bringing your palms back together. Repeat.

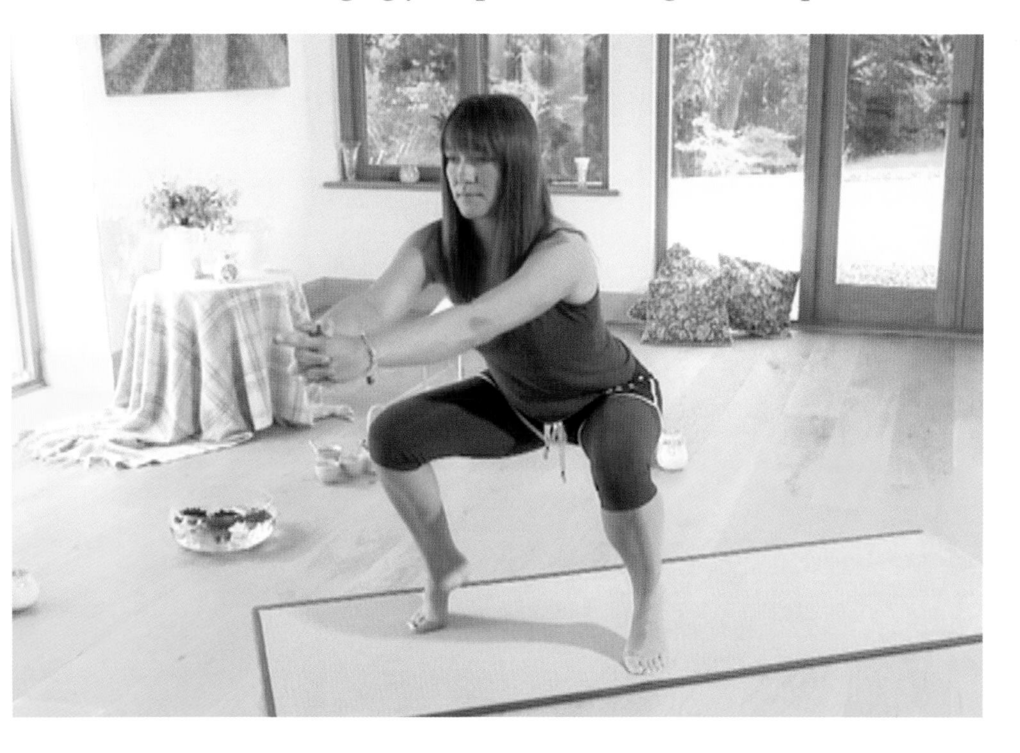

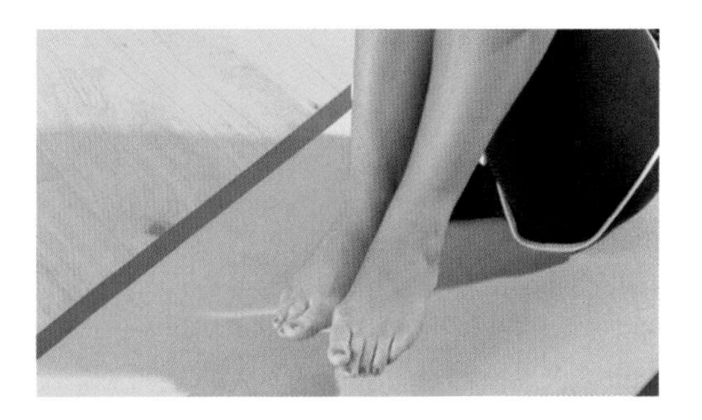

Sit with feet and knees together, hugging the knees in towards your chest, but keep the length in the back. Lift your feet up off the floor and balance and hold for around 10 seconds.

From the above position, slowly roll backwards and forwards, releasing the spine and massaging the back.

Step 1

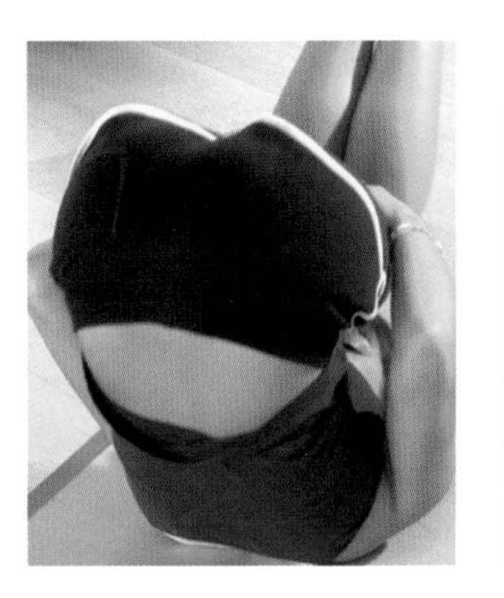

Step 2

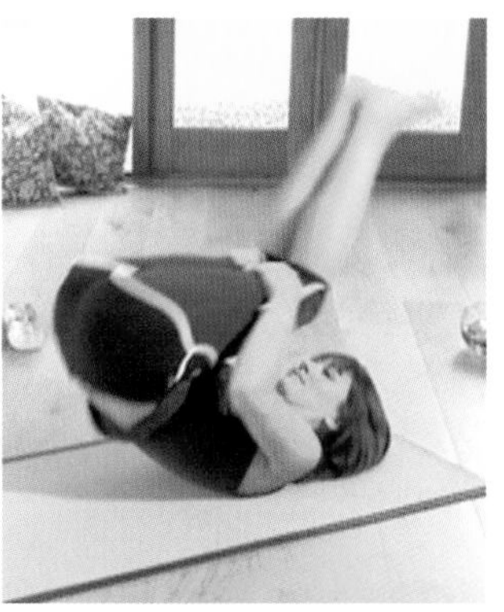

Step 3

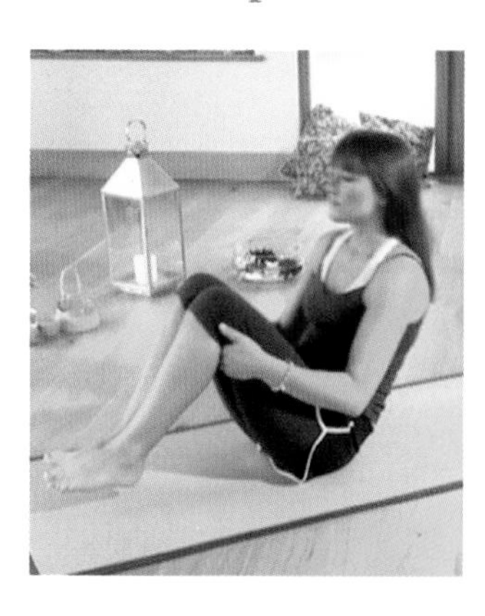

Sit with crossed legs, lift and lengthen through the spine and bring the hands back with your fingers facing away from you. Push down through the arms, and lengthen the spine.

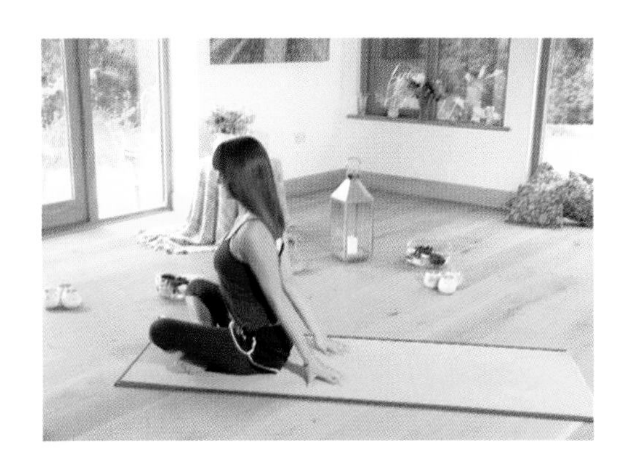

Tilt the pelvis forward and come into a forward fold, stretching the arms forward and stretching the hips. When you are at your maximum fold then release and relax into in – let the upper body, head and shoulders relax completely.

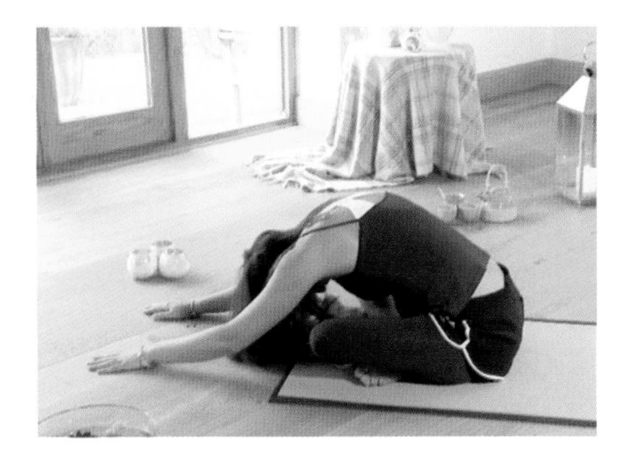

Repeat the last 2 exercises with your legs crossed the other way round.

Chapter 5

Total Body Toning With Yoga Standing Sequence

Stand with your legs about a metre apart. Put your hands on your hips, lengthen through the spine, and pull up on the thighs with your pelvis in neutral. Lift and open your chest, shoulders back and down. Engage your core to about 30% as you breath up into the chest with nice long and slow breaths.

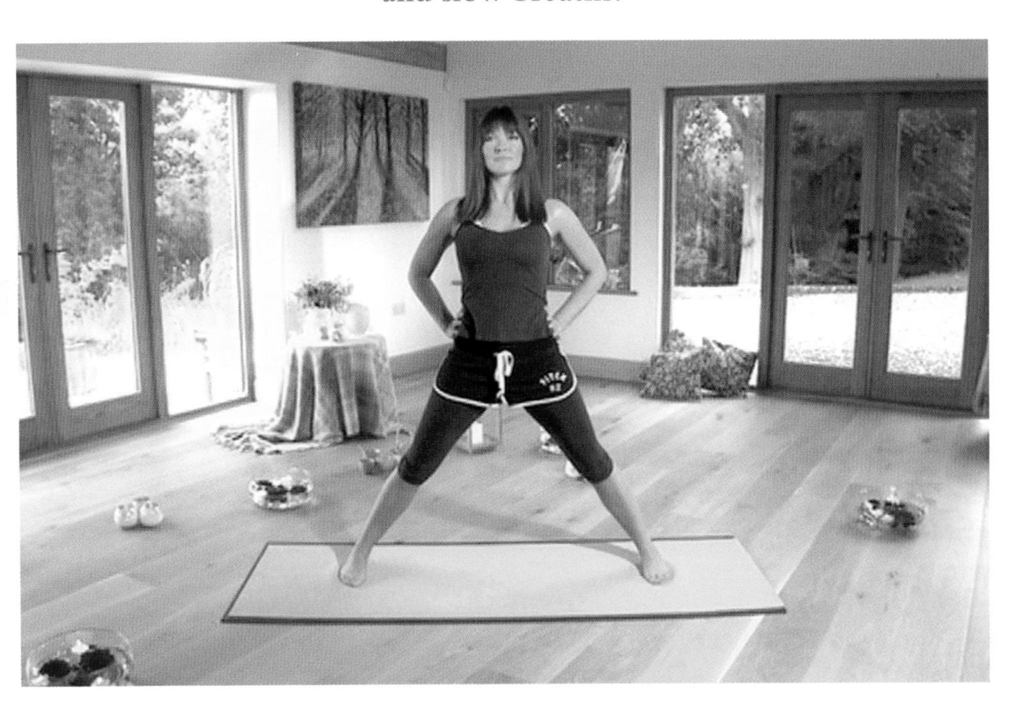

Turn sideways and put one foot forward, allowing the toes on the back foot to come to about 45 degrees. Allow the back hip to roll in as the front hip draws back. Then stretch towards your front leg, arms long.

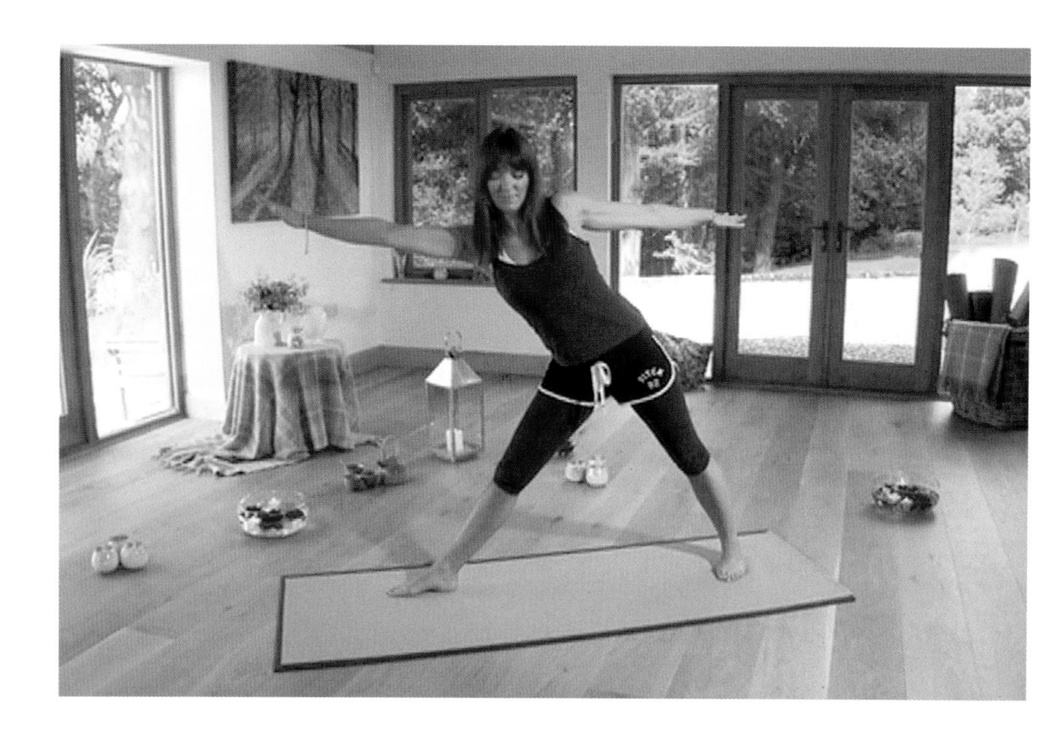

Release the forward hand down with the back hand coming up towards the ceiling, stretching out the arms and keeping your core engaged as you breath up into your chest. Keep your neck in line with your spine – chin very slightly tucked in. Hold for about 20 seconds and slowly release back up to centre then repeat with the other leg forward.

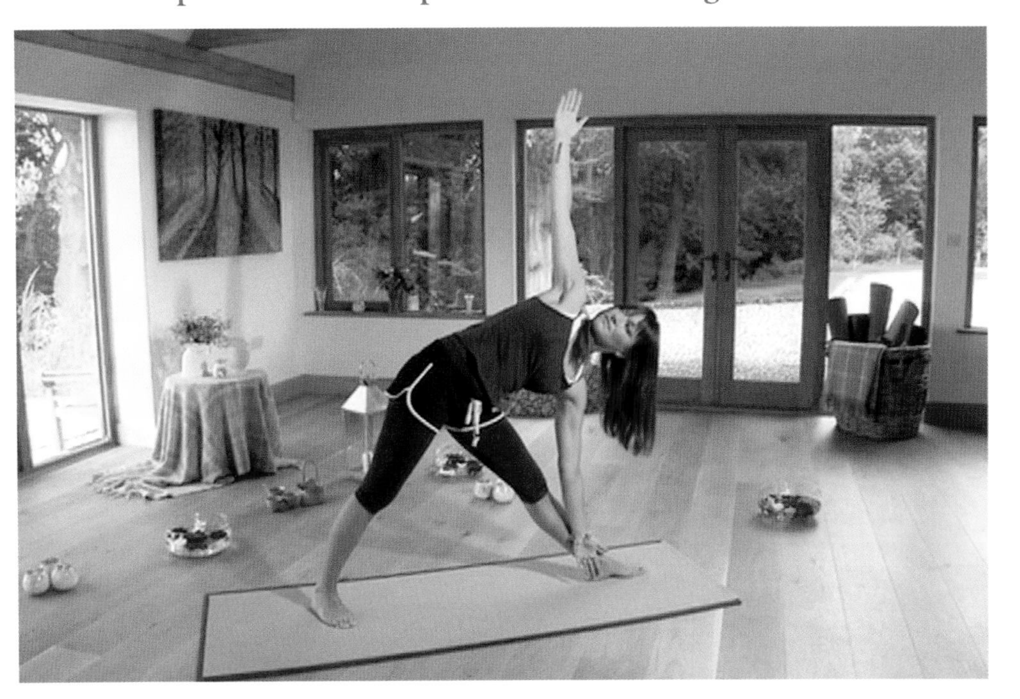

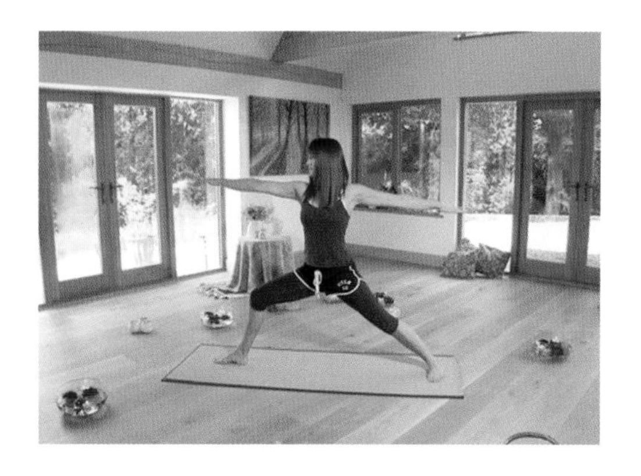

Stand with legs about one and a half metres apart, then turn to put one foot forward. Lunge forward until your knee is directly above your ankle. Straighten your arms and upper body and stretch forward and backwards until your upper body is straight. Look forward then hold the pose for about 20 seconds.

Bring your back arm onto your back leg, reaching up with the other arm and hold the stretch.

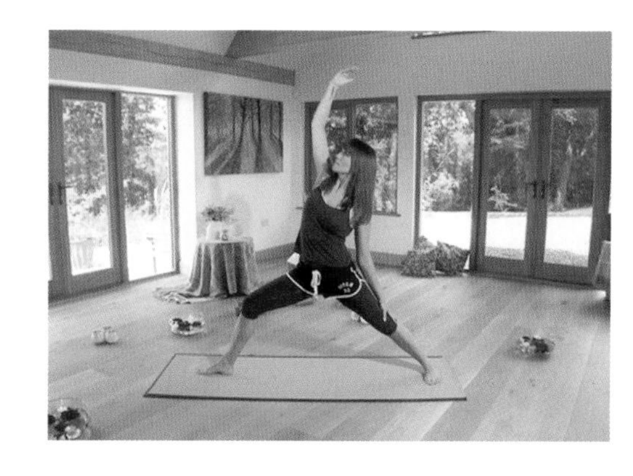

Slowly release the front elbow onto the front knee and reach up and over with the other arm, finding a straight line from the top of the hand down to the back foot. Put your front hand down to the floor if you can. Repeat the previous 3 exercises on the other leg.

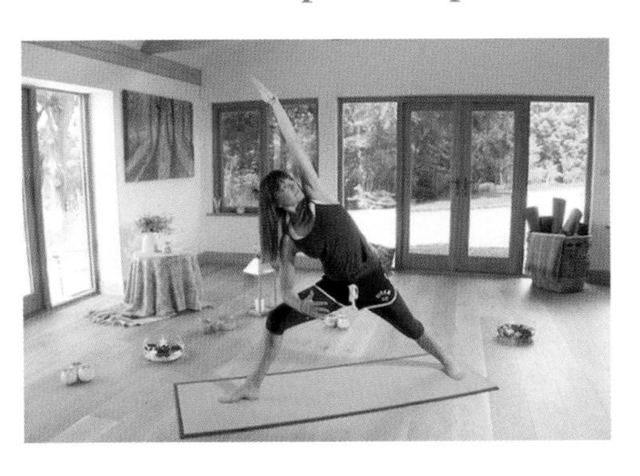

Step 1

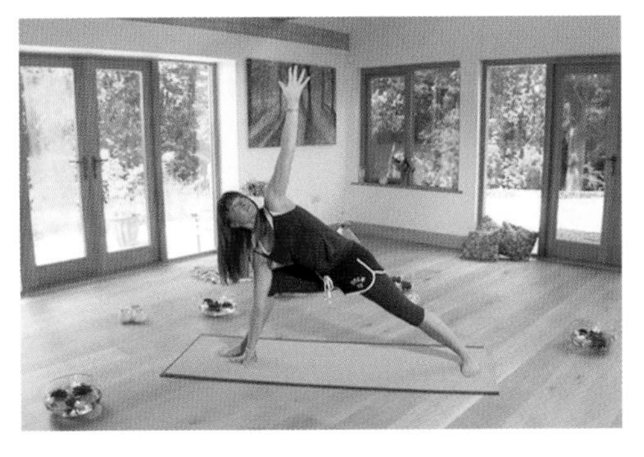

Step 2

Move into a wide legged forward bend, folding forward from the hips, letting the head relax down and breathing into the belly. Let the core relax. If you can, release your head all the way down onto the floor.

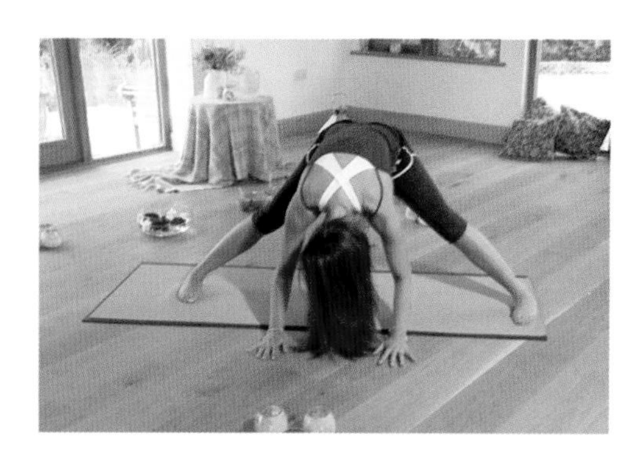

Step 1

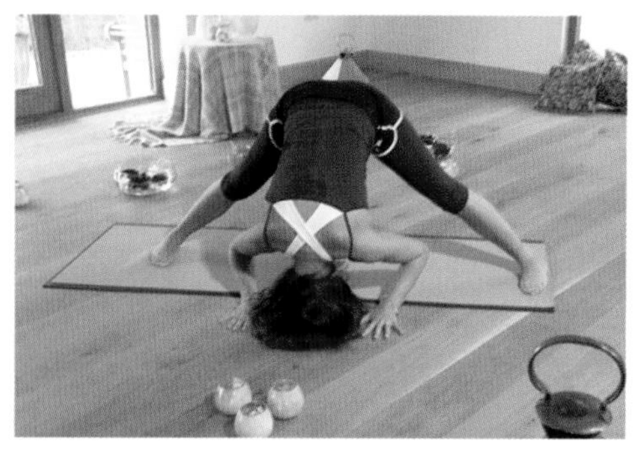

Step 2

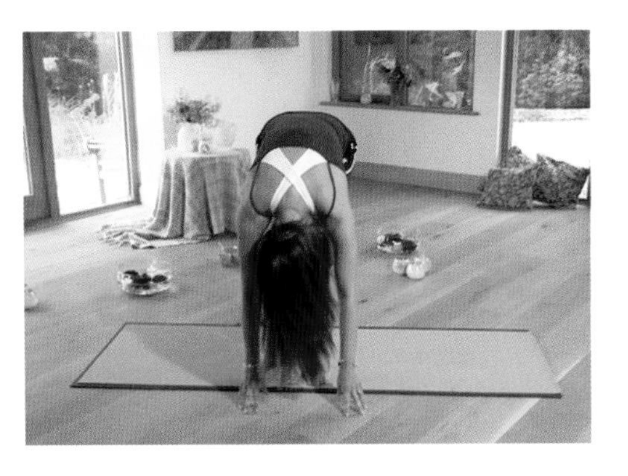

Slowly bring your feet back together, soft knees and head relaxed.

Inhale and as you exhale begin to uncurl the spine with your head coming up last.

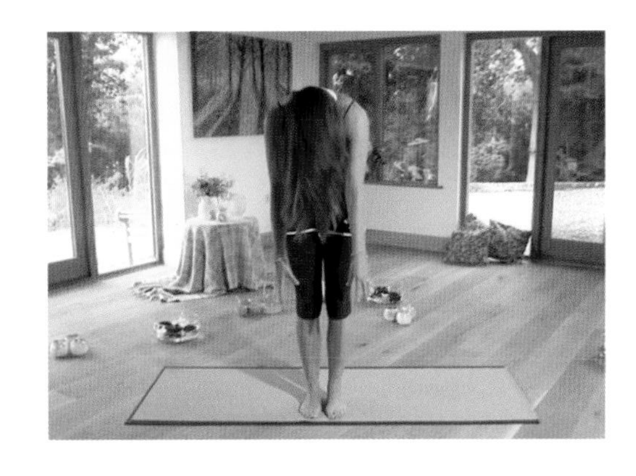

Chapter 6

Gently Opening the Hips and Shoulders

Sit in a comfortable crossed legged position, bring your right ear down to your right shoulder and let the shoulders drop down away from the ears. Keep stomach muscles completely relaxed and breath into the belly. Stretch the left arm out, stretching and then releasing for a few times. Come back to centre and repeat on the other side.

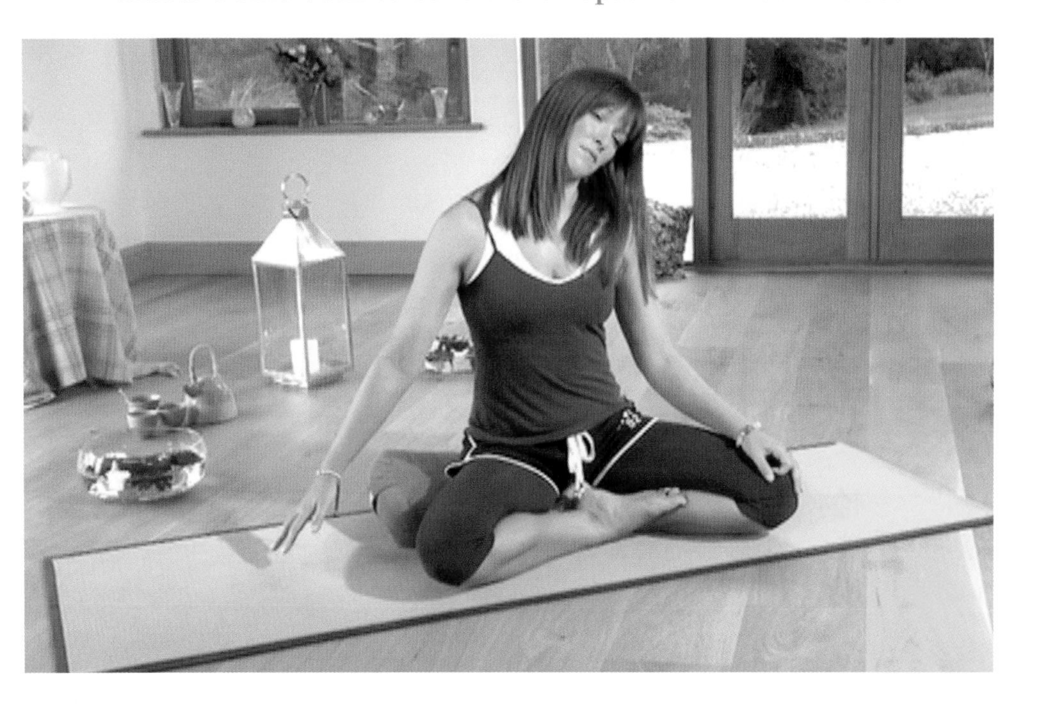

Sitting crossed legged with arms resting on your knees, gently roll your head in a semicircle from one side to the other, feeling the gentle stretch in your neck, keeping the movement soft and relaxed.

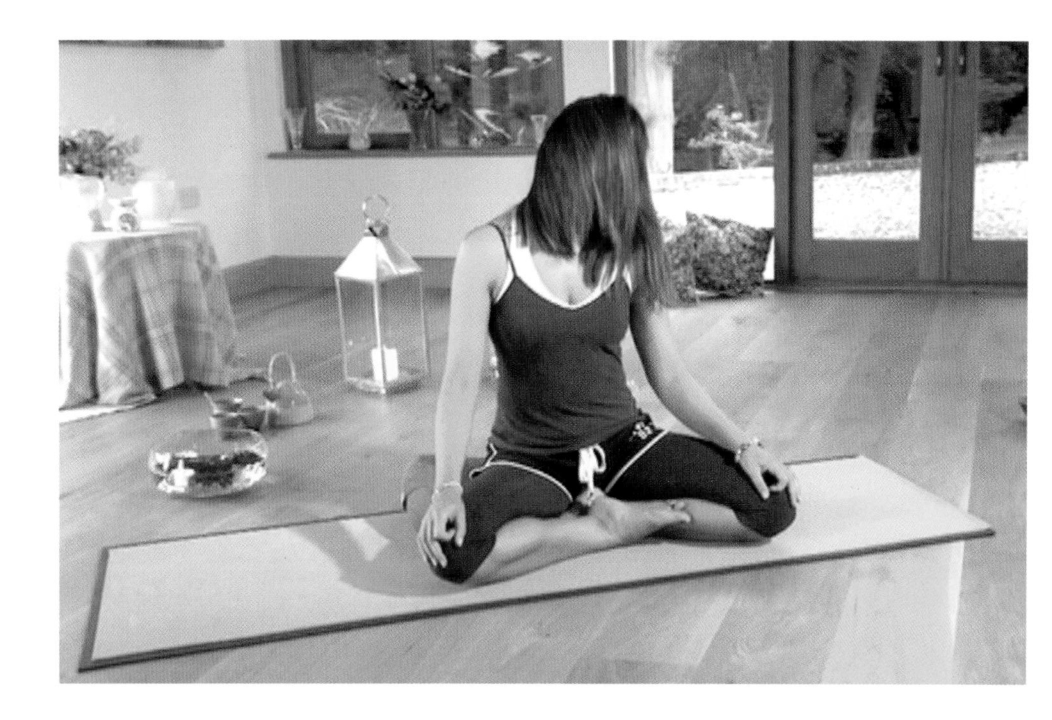

Sit up tall and raise your left arm up and wrap your right arm underneath it. If you can, bring the palms of your hands together. Let the elbows drop down slightly and let your hands come forward slightly until you start to feel a good stretch in between the shoulder blades. Repeat the other way round.

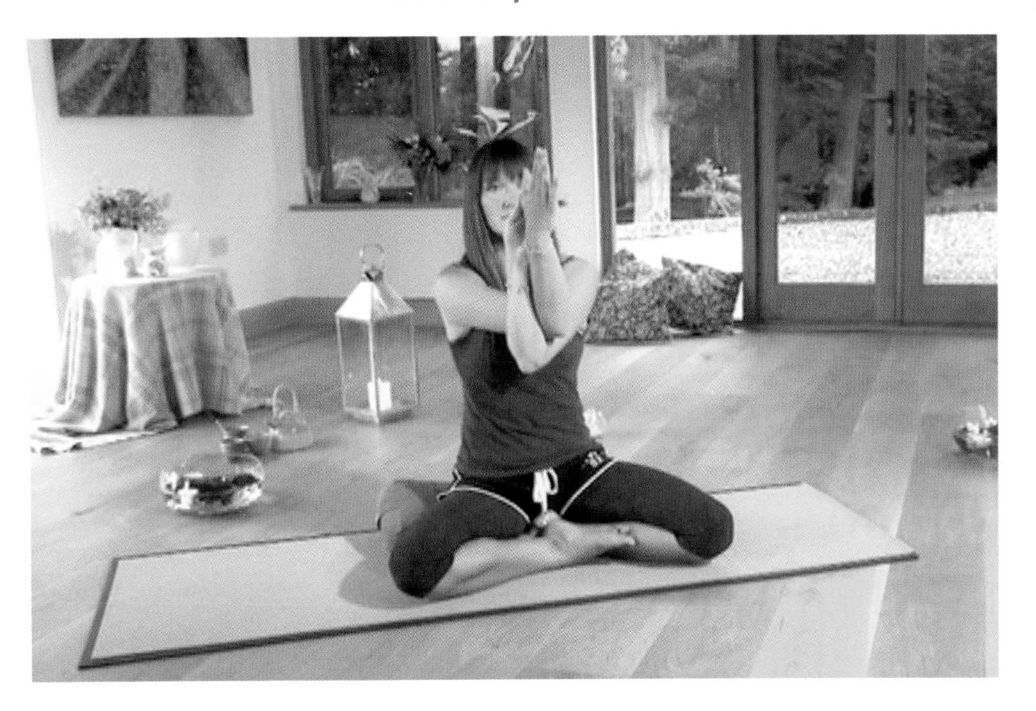

Roll the shoulders back a few times and then hunch the shoulders right up, then letting them drop. Repeat twice more.

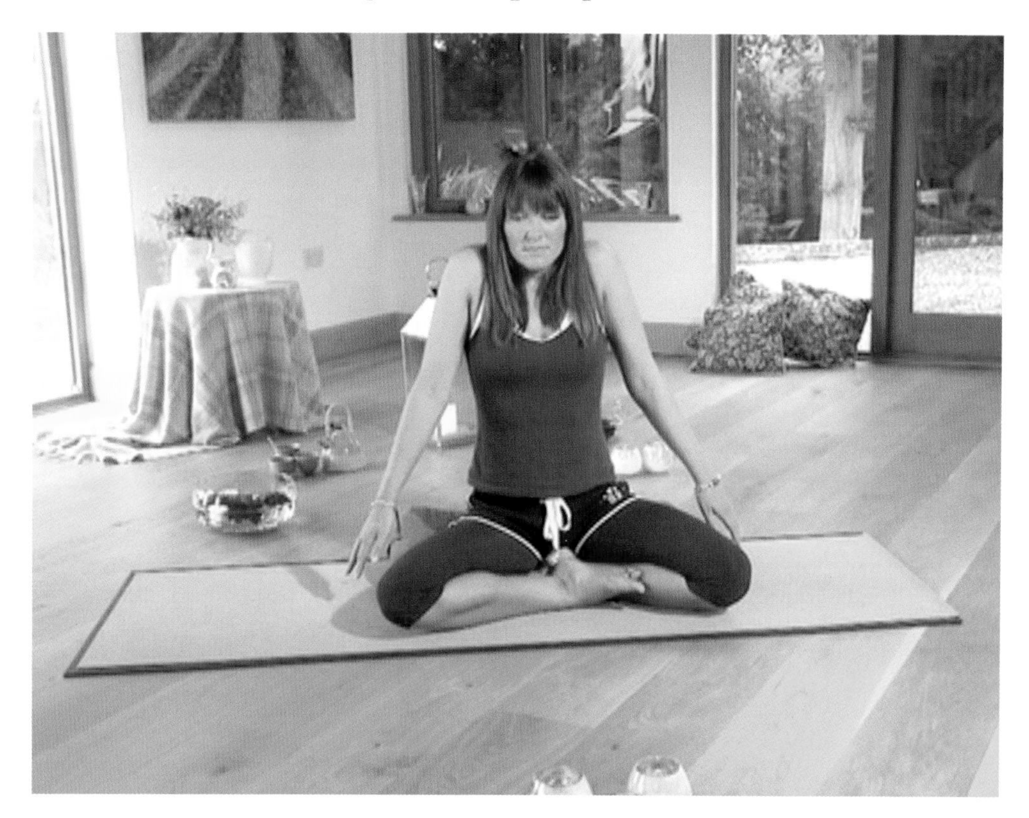

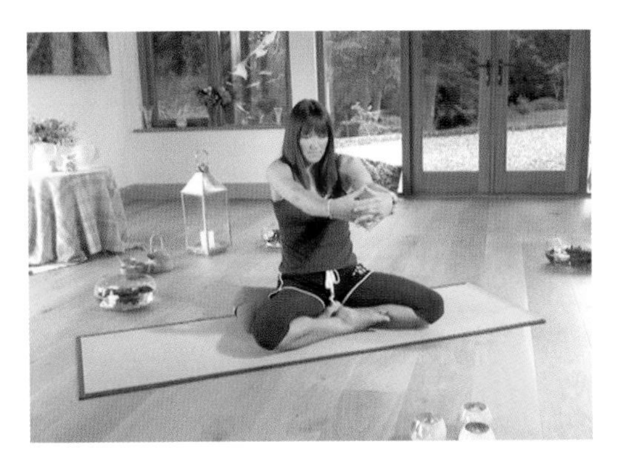

Interlace your hands and push your arms forward and sink back stretching out your upper back.

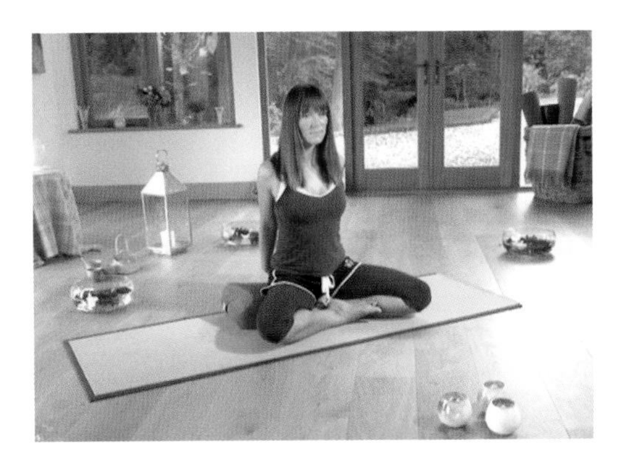

Interlace your hands behind your back and squeeze your shoulder blades back.

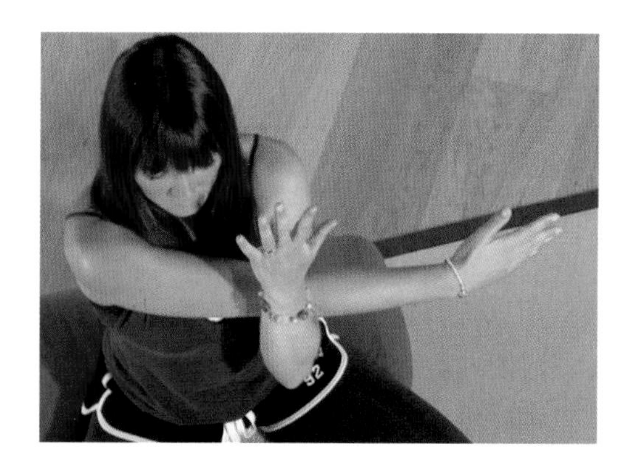

Bring your left arm across the body, easing it back with the right and repeat on the other side.

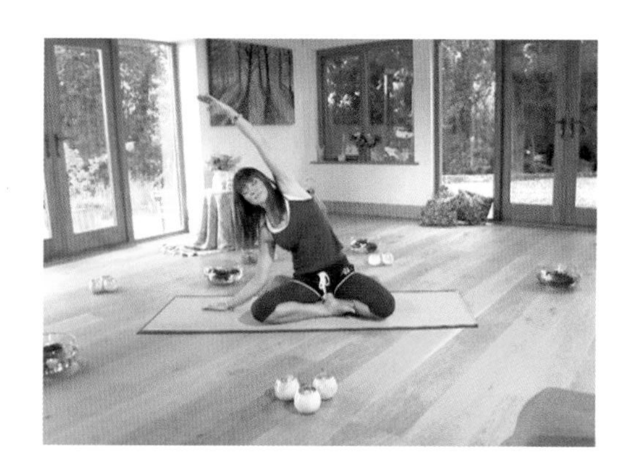

Stretch over to one side and then over to the other.

Lie with your knees bent and your feet flat on the floor. Bring the right foot in front of the left knee and then lift the left leg up off the floor. Slide your hands in between the gap in your legs, easing the knee back towards you and hold. Keep your neck and shoulders relaxed. Slowly release and repeat on the other side.

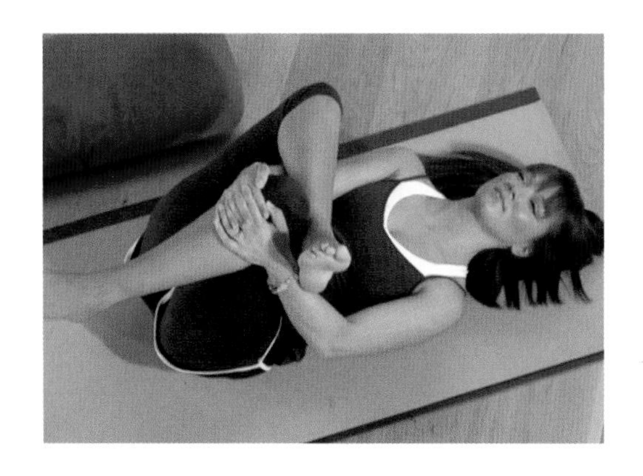

Hug your knees in and then begin to circle the knees around by drawing them in towards you and then away from you. Then do it in the opposite direction.

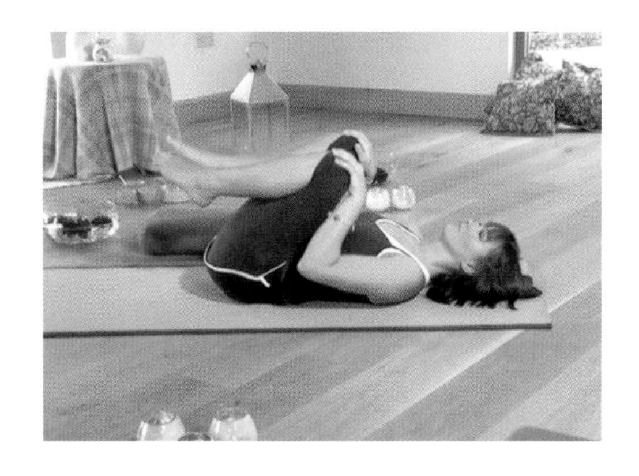

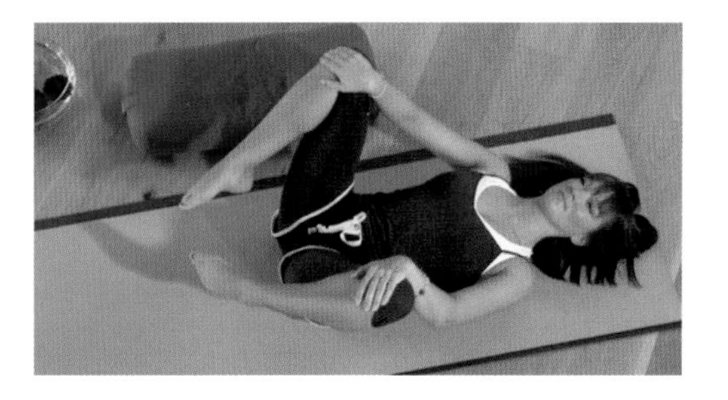

Draw the knees out wide and rest your hands on the inside of the knees and circle your feet from your ankles.

Draw one knee in towards you, then straighten the leg, holding behind the back of the leg down towards the ankle. If that feels ok then lift the head up to stretch the leg a little more deeply. Draw the knee in and then out to the side a little, avoiding the rib cage, and release down.

Step 1

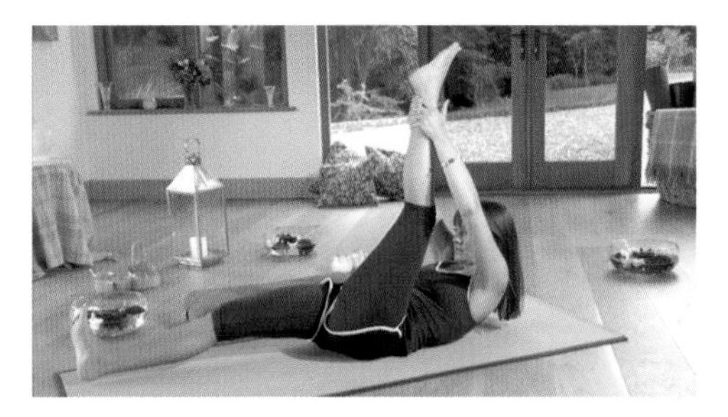

Step 2

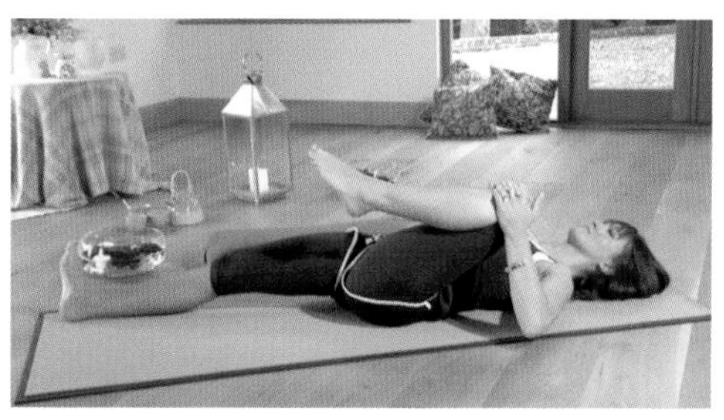

Repeat the previous 2 exercises on the other side.

Hug both knees in and hold.

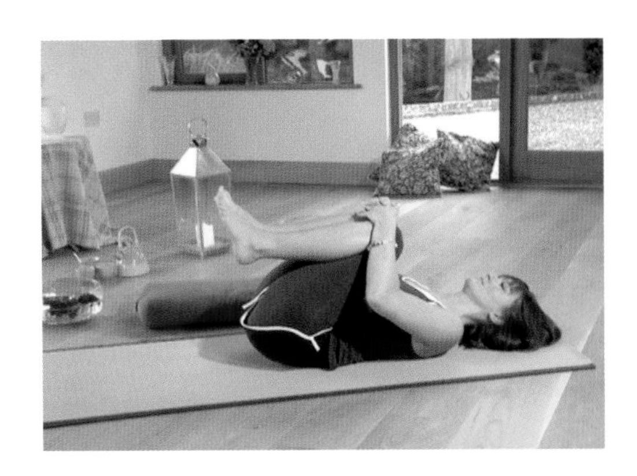

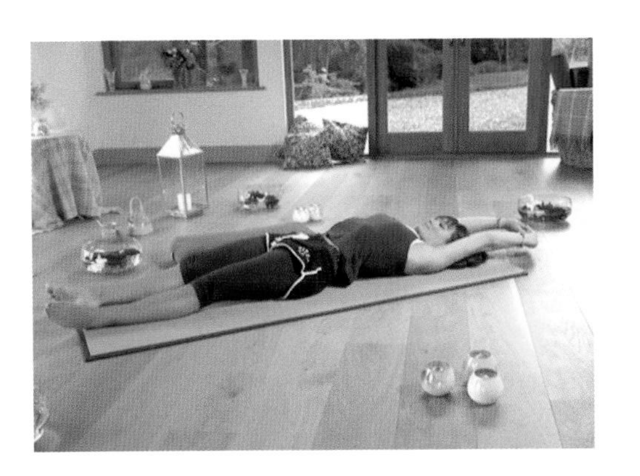

Lie long and bring the arms back behind you coming into a full body stretch, reaching through the fingers and toes. Interlace your hands and stretch through them and the feet.

Lie comfortably on the floor with your arms by your side and relaxed. Just feel the whole body relaxing.

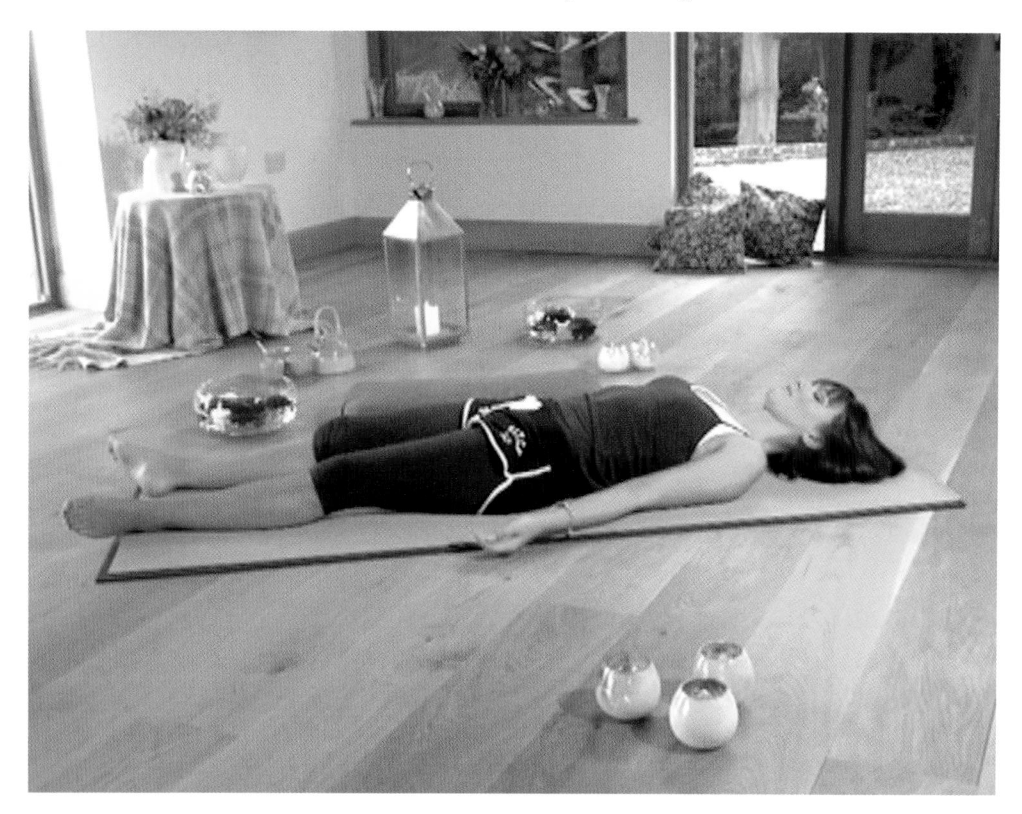

Chapter 7

Blissful Relaxation

Lie in a comfortable position, flex the feet back towards you and squeeze the legs to ease out any tension in the body and then release. Repeat a few times. Then squeeze the hips and the buttocks as much as you can for a few seconds and then release. Repeat a few times. Sink the lower back down to the floor and squeeze the stomach muscles, hold, then release it all. Repeat a few times.

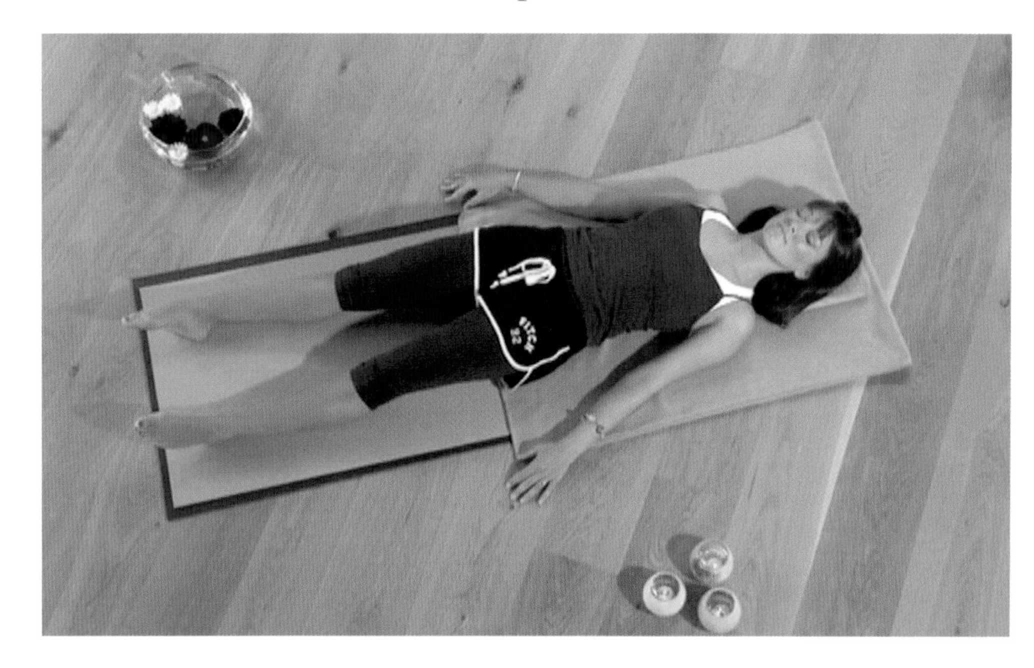

Hunch the shoulders up around the ears, squeezing right the way up and then release.

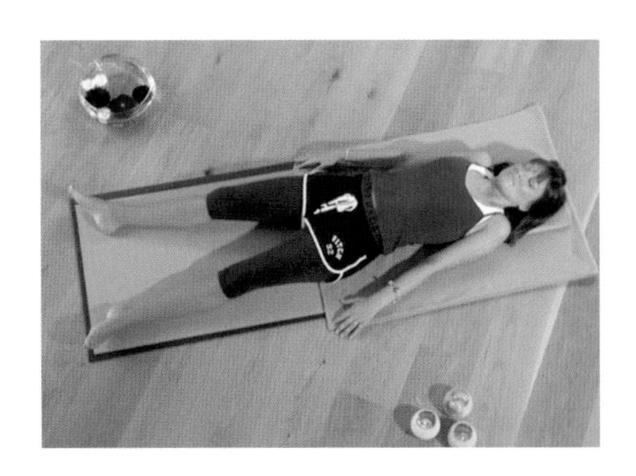

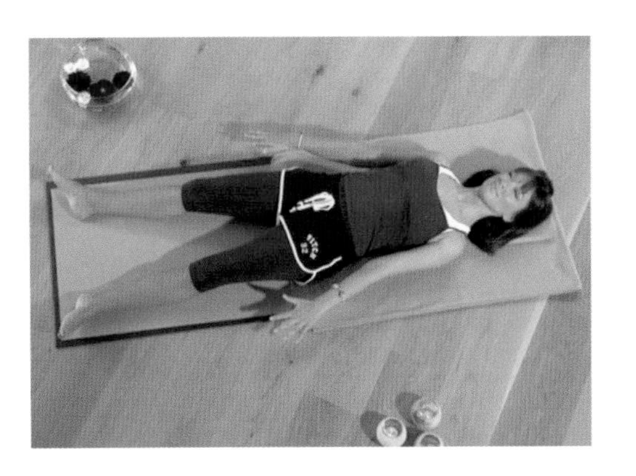

Reach with your arms down beside you, stretching through the fingers and then release.

Tuck the chin into the neck and squeeze the neck muscles, hold, and release.

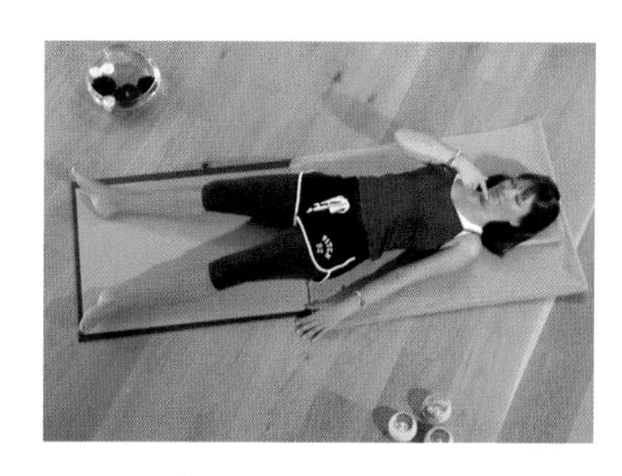

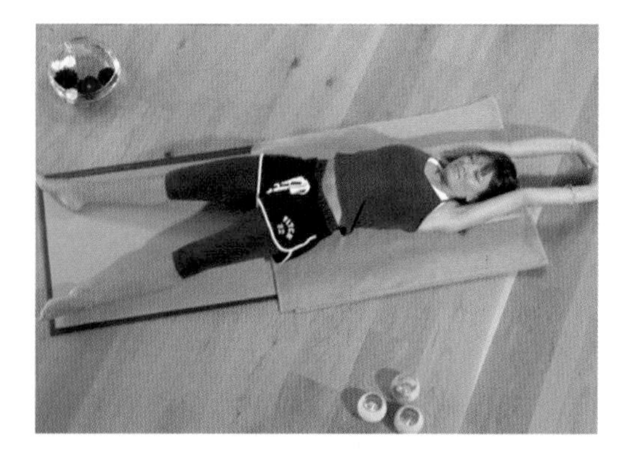

Bring the arms back behind the head, moving into a full body stretch, reaching through the fingers, hold, and release.

Lie in a comfortable position and relax absolutely everything from your tongue to your toes. Every time you exhale your body should relax even further as you breath out any tension in your body. Focus on relaxing every part of your body for at least 5 minutes, particularly focusing on any parts of your body where you still feel any tension. Say to yourself, 'my whole body is completely relaxed' and 'my mind is completely relaxed'.

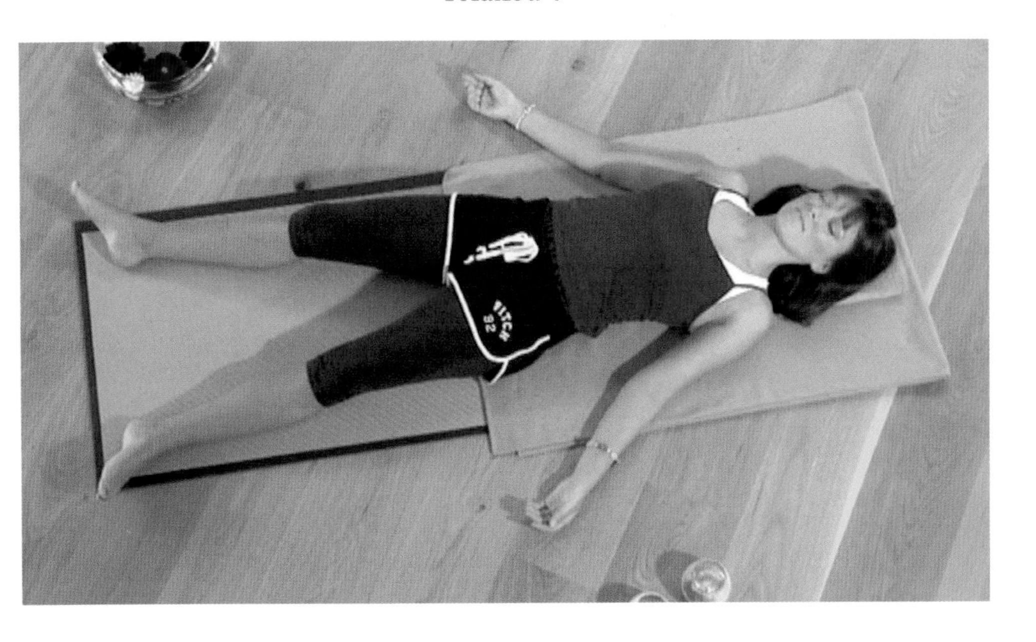

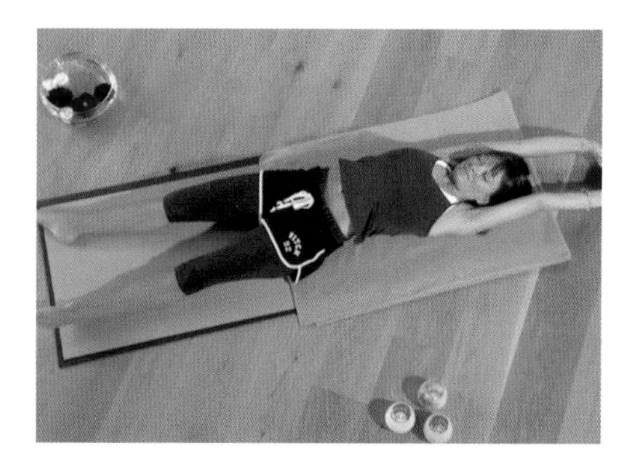

Gradually bring your awareness back to the surface. Start gently circling your feet and bring the arms back behind the head coming into a full body stretch.

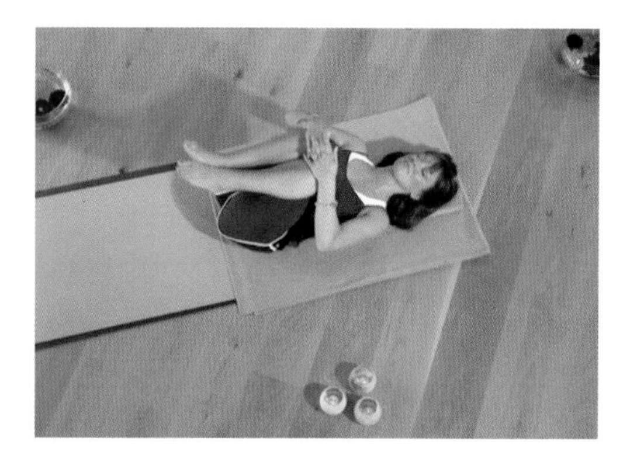

Draw the knees in, stretching out the lower back.

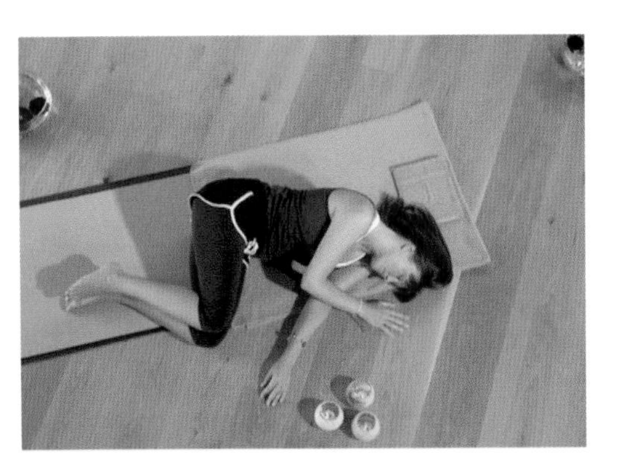

Roll onto one side and just rest there for a few seconds.

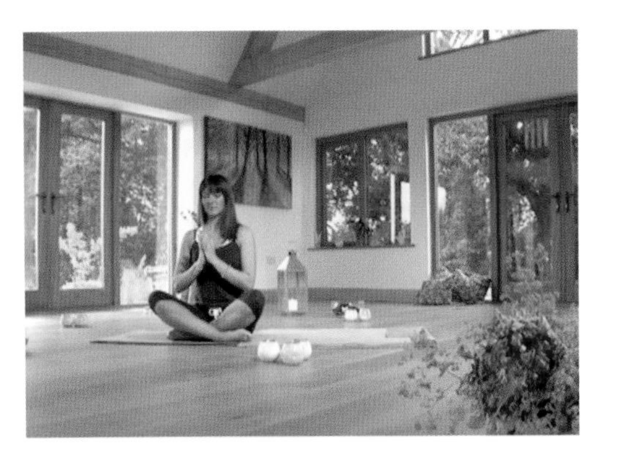

Slowly come back to sitting with legs crossed and hands to your hearts centre.

Design and artwork by Scott Giarnese

Published by Demand Media Limited

Publishers Jason Fenwick & Jules Gammond

Written by Michelle Brachet